Critical Appraisal Skills for Healthcare Students

Critical Appraisal Skills for Healthcare Students

A Practical Guide to Writing Evidence-based Practice Assignments

Charlotte J. Whiffin
University of Derby, Derby, UK

Donna Barnes
University of Derby, Derby, UK

Lorraine Henshaw
University of Salford, Manchester, UK

Illustrations by
Brandon Smith

WILEY Blackwell

This edition first published 2024
© 2024 John Wiley & Sons Ltd

The right of Charlotte J. Whiffin, Donna Barnes, and Lorraine Henshaw to be identified as the authors of this work has been asserted in accordance with law.

Registered Offices
John Wiley & Sons, Inc., 111 River Street, Hoboken, NJ 07030, USA
John Wiley & Sons Ltd, The Atrium, Southern Gate, Chichester, West Sussex, PO19 8SQ, UK

For details of our global editorial offices, customer services, and more information about Wiley products visit us at www.wiley.com.

Wiley also publishes its books in a variety of electronic formats and by print-on-demand. Some content that appears in standard print versions of this book may not be available in other formats.

Library of Congress Cataloging-in-Publication Data Applied for:

Paperback ISBN: 9781119722816
ePDF: 9781119722892
ePUB: 9781119722847

Cover Design: Wiley
Cover Image: © Jacob Lund/Shutterstock

Set in 10.5/13pt STIXTwoText by Straive, Pondicherry, India
Printed and bound by CPI Group (UK) Ltd, Croydon, CR0 4YY
C9781119722816_040324

For David, Emily, Grace, and Mum x

For my friends x

For Toby, Niamh and Leo xx

... and for all our students

Quality is not an act, it is a habit.
Aristotle

All great achievements require time.
Maya Angelou

The important thing is not to stop questioning. Curiosity has its own reason for existing.
Albert Einstein

Nothing in life is to be feared. It is only to be understood.
Marie Curie

Nothing is impossible, I do nothing every day.
Winnie the Pooh

Contents

Foreword

Dr Andrew Dainty
Senior Lecturer in Pre-Qualifying Health Care, University of Derby, UK

Every year, thousands of healthcare students are faced with the seemingly mammoth task of mastering critical appraisal skills, and developing the knowledge and skills required to apply them to research used to underpin professional healthcare practice. In fact, for some, the very mention of the word research brings about apprehension and feelings of general anxiety. If this applies to you, then thankfully you have come to the right place. The authors of this book are experts in helping students grasp fundamental critical appraisal skills, and so *Critical Appraisal Skills for Healthcare Students* came to fruition because of this passion.

Evidence-based practice is ultimately about ensuring that people receiving care have access to the most appropriate interventions, underpinned by robust scientific evidence. While it is true that clinicians will not always be able to appraise individual research studies themselves, understanding the concepts behind appraisal is essential for one to grasp the premise behind how evidence-based guidelines are formed. Despite the need for meticulous appraisal, research studies are seldom rejected outright, and appraisal takes place to arrive at a balanced decision based on the facts and potential sources of bias. This results in the identification of certain strengths and limitations. In fact, all research has both, but even the most poorly designed of studies can often have some element of usefulness.

Throughout the following chapters the authors will take you on a journey, and hopefully this will help to demystify some aspects of critical thinking and appraisal that are frequently encountered by healthcare students. If you are struggling with these topics and you have been looking for a good place to start, then Part 1 is all about some of the fundamental aspects of locating and identifying different types of research.

Locating research, identifying the different types of research, and determining its potential usefulness can often be tricky. This book provides information to save time and energy searching for studies that are relevant to the task at hand. Once you have some understanding of the fundamentals of research evidence, Part 2 will provide you with information that can be used to develop critical thinking and will show you how to apply this appraisal to your practice. The truth is that there is no perfect choice of methods, because all types of research have strengths and limitations.

This book explores the process of developing critical writing skills and is intended to help you to write for academic assessments. The authors cover the formulation of coherent and logical argument based on consideration of the merits and limitations of research. The book is about the skills and knowledge needed to aid you in the process of appraisal, the basis of which should enable you to have a good understanding of what research is all about, and how to judge its worth. Once developed, these skills will serve you well for the rest of your career in healthcare, and this book is a good foundation on which to base your continual professional development related to research.

Preface

For over a decade, we have had the pleasure of teaching healthcare students about research and the art of critical appraisal. Many students arrive at their research modules feeling overwhelmed and intimidated about what lies ahead. Helping students to understand research, while watching their enthusiasm and confidence grow, has been a highlight of our teaching careers. This is especially true when students tell us at the end of the module that they have 'secretly' grown to enjoy research!

While it's important to point out that not all students start with a negative perception of research, we understand why some do. The use of research is often invisible or undervalued in practice. It also has a reputation for being boring and requiring superhuman boffin powers to understand it. We have loved smashing these myths during our teaching, by encouraging lively classroom debates about controversial clinical evidence and entertaining students with our favourite research jokes (what do you mean you didn't know there were any research jokes?).

However, we found that problems arose after class, when students started to work on their assignments and were faced with some serious textbooks. These were often either too detailed for those needing to appraise a study rather than conduct one, or too basic for getting to grips with the complexities of evidence-based practice. Students also said they struggled to find resources to help them write about research and make critical points about studies in an informed and analytical way.

So our aim was to create a book that met these needs: not too advanced, not too basic, not too theoretical, and not too lightweight. Instead, like Goldilocks' perfect porridge, we aimed for something 'just right'.

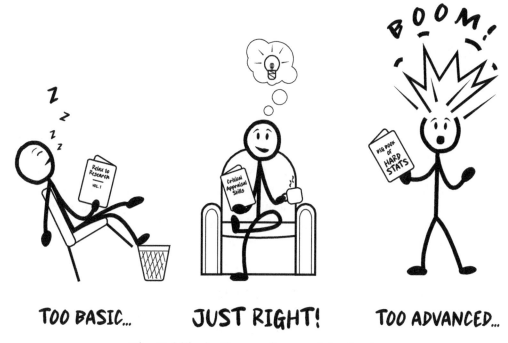

The Goldilocks theory of research textbooks

While it would be lovely to think that this book will inspire students to conduct their own research, we wanted to create a book that helps students more practically with the thing that is most important to them when they start a research module – to pass the assignment! We also wanted to create a book that is a little more fun, so that learning about research is enjoyable rather than unbearable.

Lastly, we wanted to be guided by those who had started us on this journey, by sharing their anxieties and insecurities with us, and inspiring us to develop creative research teaching practice. So this book was created *with students, for students*, and we hope it gives you all the tools you need to succeed!

Charlotte (Charlie) Whiffin RN PhD
Donna Barnes RN PhD
Lorraine Henshaw RN DProf

Acknowledgements

We would like to thank Naila Dracup, information specialist, who reviewed Chapter 4 on locating evidence and provided additional advice and guidance on the content. This just goes to show how valuable it is to work with a librarian!

We would also like to thank all the students who contributed to this book. The book is written with students, for students, and we hope your insights and reflections will help others both survive and thrive in their evidence-based practice and research modules in the future.

Danielle Anderson
Rebecca Baxter
Franzer Baldove
Jaclyn Beardmore
Katie Cockayne
Carly Forrester
Lucy Gee
Jodie Hinchliffe
Kelly Kemp
Alasdair MacDonald
Ellis Mack
Catia Neiva
Georgina Noble
Beth Orton
Rosamund Pocklington
Benjamin Powell-Jones
Amy Pyrek-Wright
Lucy Stanway
Naomi Somers
Laura Taylor
Colleen Thompson
Sylvie Umutoni
Terri Wilson
Alan Wilton

PART I

FINDING YOUR WAY AROUND!

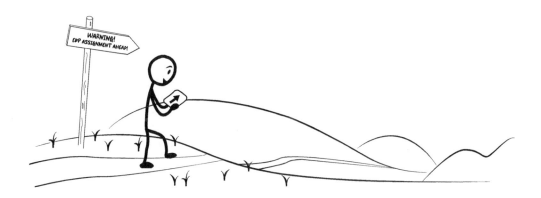

CHAPTER 1

Introduction to Using This Book

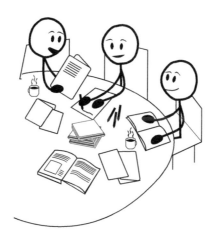

1.1 INTRODUCTION

Classic – a book which people praise and don't read.

Mark Twain

There are plenty of 'classic' research texts and all have their place in the learning journey. But do we ever really 'read' research textbooks? Perhaps some people do, but

Critical Appraisal Skills for Healthcare Students: A Practical Guide to Writing Evidence-based Practice Assignments, First Edition. Charlotte J. Whiffin, Donna Barnes, and Lorraine Henshaw.

it is more likely that we move from book to book, acquiring pieces of information that we then put together like a jigsaw puzzle in an assignment. Our aim for this book is that its sections can be dipped into and out of to suit your learning needs. But we also want it to be a book that can be read easily from cover to cover and hopefully enjoyed. So, fingers crossed!

1.2   WHO IS THE BOOK FOR?

This book is primarily aimed at academic level 5 healthcare students who need to complete critical appraisal assignments of primary research. However, the content is also suitable for academic level 4 or 6 assignments on the concept of evidence-based practice (EBP), using research evidence for healthcare, and extended litera-ture reviews.

The book is designed to support students with applying their learning about research and EBP to written assignments and developing their academic writing skills. These skills can be used for non-research assignments too, since they support students to locate, understand, and use research evidence on any healthcare topic.

1.3   WHAT IS IN THIS BOOK?

Throughout the book you will follow our **EBP process for academic assessment** (Figure 1.1). Our model broadly follows the traditional EBP process (more on this in Chapter 2), but we have added a few stages so you can apply it more easily to your academic work. Our process will support you to work through each stage in a logical order and relate these to the chapter content. However, each stage may be applied differently within the context of your specific assessment, so always check your assignment brief to be sure.

In each chapter there are several features to support your learning and help you to navigate your way through the content (see Table 1.1). Through these we highlight key content, encourage active engagement and consolidation, and provide worked examples.

In addition to the features listed in Table 1.1, we have also separated the book into two distinct parts. **Part 1** explains what you need to know before you conduct critical appraisal activities for academic assessments. **Part 2** then gives you the tools to appraise research and write about this appraisal to meet level 5 criteria.

1.3.1   Part 1: Finding Your Way Around!

In this first chapter, 'Introduction to Using This Book', we do exactly that! We explain who the book was written for and what makes it unique. We will also explain how to use this book to get the most out of the contents.

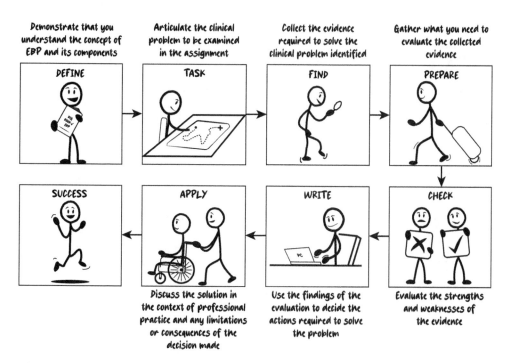

FIGURE 1.1   The EBP process for academic assessment.

Chapter 2, 'Professional Practice and the Mandate for Evidence-based Practice', takes a necessary look at the relevance of EBP to the healthcare profession and why so many professional programmes include assignments based on appraisal activities. We review definitions, models, hierarchies, and criticisms of this approach to patient care.

Chapter 3, 'The Task at Hand', asks you to take a closer look at your learning outcomes and assignment briefs to make sure you are well prepared.

Chapter 4, 'Locating and Identifying Research', aims to give you the skills to find good-quality healthcare evidence. Although some of you will have been given a research study to appraise for the assessment, some of you will need to locate your own. Either way, this chapter will support you to develop the searching skills that are fundamental for evidence-based practice and for level 6 assignments that require you to conduct a literature review.

Chapter 5, 'Preparing the Ground for Appraisal', encourages you to be sure that you have a primary research paper for appraisal, that you are able to navigate your way around it, and gives you some much-needed strategies and tips for successfully reading research evidence.

1.3.2   Part 2: Digging in the Detail!

Chapter 6, 'Critical Appraisal', starts you off on the journey to critical appraisal of primary research. The chapter first ensures that you know what type of research you

TABLE 1.1   Features in this book.

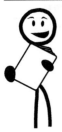

Five minutes with. . .. are personal reflections that have been contributed by our students and are about how they felt during their EBP/research modules, how they completed the module tasks and wrote their assignments, and any tips and tricks they feel you may benefit from.

Assignment tips offer some useful suggestions for how you may use the chapter content in your assignment.

Research essentials provide definitions or explanations of key terms or concepts that you may not be familiar with, but are important to understand for critically appraising research.

Explore it boxes give an opportunity to investigate additional resources that will extend your understanding of the chapter content.

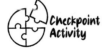

Checkpoint activities offer you a chance to engage more actively with the content, to check your understanding and encourage deeper learning.

Assignment examples towards the end of most chapters are small snippets of real students' work to illustrate how students have written about the chapter content in their level 5 assignments. Be warned! Don't copy these and paste them into assignments. You could be accused of plagiarism or, worse, professional misconduct. Instead, use the examples to help you develop your own academic writing style.

TABLE 1.1   (Continued)

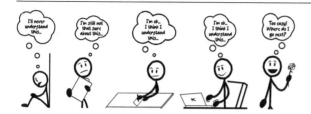

End-of-chapter checkpoints at the end of each chapter give you a way of checking your understanding of the chapter content. By completing a checkpoint you will have a good sense of what you know about the topic, and what you don't. Therefore, these checklists may increase your confidence in what you know and will identify areas where you would benefit from further learning.

KEY FACTS

Key facts sheets at the end of Chapter 7, 'Appraising Quantitative Research', and Chapter 8, 'Appraising Qualitative Research', provide quick summaries of specific research designs so you can focus on the important issues associated with these. Each facts sheet includes our EDECA appraisal considerations (Ethics, Design, Enrol, Collect, Analyse) that explain what to look out for in these studies.

have so that you can use the subsequent chapters appropriately. To help you in this task, we introduce some fundamental characteristics of qualitative, quantitative, and mixed methods research. We then focus in on appraisal, what this really means, and what tools are available to help you.

Chapter 7, 'Appraising Quantitative Research', and Chapter 8, 'Appraising Qualitative Research', address the appraisal of quantitative and qualitative research, respectively, enabling you to focus in on the issues that are most relevant to your chosen study. First, we review typical aims and methods associated with each research type and provide a 'key facts sheet' for each of the most common research designs associated with quantitative and qualitative approaches. As there is no mixed methods chapter in this book, for reasons we will explain later, we have included a mixed methods fact sheet as an appendix for those who may find this useful.

Chapter 9, 'Writing Up Your Research Appraisal', shows you how to incorporate research appraisal into a written level 5 assignment. We tackle the challenging issue of differentiating between descriptive and analytical writing styles, and how you can demonstrate your informed understanding of research quality within your assignment. We achieve this through our DJES tool, 'Describe–Evaluate–Justify–Support', and provide worked examples so that you can demonstrate your ability to critically appraise research while also meeting level 5 academic criteria.

Chapter 10, 'Appraisal in Context', is the final chapter, in which we come full circle back to the concept of EBP. Here we explain the end goal of locating and appraising evidence, which is to apply the knowledge in a professional healthcare context. We consider some aspects that inhibit the use of evidence in practice as well as some strategies for facilitating it. We close with some final words of wisdom.

1.4   CHAPTER SUMMARY

In this short first chapter we have introduced this book and described its contents. We have explained who we had in mind when we wrote the book and how to get the best from it. Now it's time to buckle up and get ready for evidence-based practice and the journey through critical appraisal to writing, and passing, your assignment!

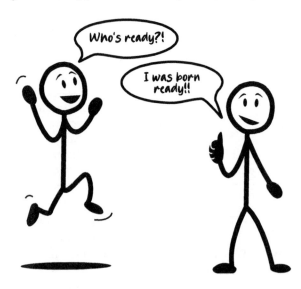

CHAPTER 2

Professional Practice and the Mandate for Evidence-based Practice

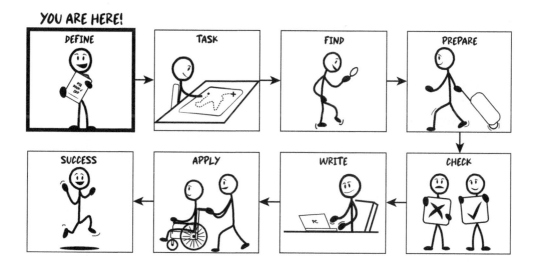

FIVE THINGS TO LEARN FROM THIS CHAPTER

1. Evidence-based practice (EBP) originated from evidence-based medicine (EBM), which advocates a scientific approach to practice.
2. EBP consists of three interrelated parts: evidence; expertise; patients.

Critical Appraisal Skills for Healthcare Students: A Practical Guide to Writing Evidence-based Practice Assignments, First Edition. Charlotte J. Whiffin, Donna Barnes, and Lorraine Henshaw.
© 2024 John Wiley & Sons Ltd. Published 2024 by John Wiley & Sons Ltd.

3. EBP is a stepped process involving asking questions; locating the evidence; appraising the evidence; integrating the evidence; and evaluating the outcomes.

4. Hierarchies of evidence illustrate the weighting given to different types of evidence in solving clinical problems.

5. There are limitations and criticisms relating to EBP that must be addressed when considering effective ways to use evidence for practice.

FIVE MINUTES WITH SARA, MIDWIFERY STUDENT

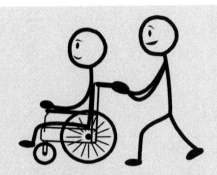

Do you see evidence being used in practice?
I think evidence is used in practice, but I do not always think that people know the reason behind why they are using it fully. Sometimes it seems like we as students are more aware of the evidence base on an issue than the registered staff who have been in practice a long time.

It takes a long time for evidence to filter through to practice, because of the EBP process. It also takes a lot of organisational support. COVID was a good example of how changes can be implemented quickly when everyone is on board and supporting it. Otherwise, it can take years to change the existing culture of the ward. The other issues are just the current pressures – no staff, no time.

In what assignment did you have to write about EBP?
I've written about EBP several times during my programme. Specifically, a couple of appraisal assignments and now my dissertation. However, EBP has been incorporated in most assignments throughout the course, particularly in year 2.

What advice would you give to students learning about EBP for the first time?
I think it's helpful to motivate yourself, for example thinking about the benefits to your own practice and your future working

life. When you understand evidence you can understand the reasons for certain changes in practice and it can help you to keep up with developments. Healthcare is so dynamic, and things are always changing. You need to be able to adapt.

You should read the materials given and attend classroom lessons as we are all different types of learners. Ask questions, remember there are 'no silly questions!' EBP will be part of your future careers and it will be required on a daily basis. This reinforces the importance of understanding EBP so it can be put into practice in order to provide safe and quality care.

2.1   INTRODUCTION

In this chapter we will introduce you to the concept of evidence-based practice, which is more commonly known by its abbreviation, EBP. This may be something you are familiar with already or just starting to learn about, but what does it actually mean for you, the patients you care for, and the profession you are joining? This chapter will help you to understand how EBP can benefit your professional practice and the care you provide, but will also explain its complexities and how they can be discussed in your EBP assignments.

The chapter begins by explaining the relevance of EBP for healthcare professions and why research assignments are so commonly found in pre-registration healthcare programmes. The chapter then explores the historical development of the EBP movement, the evolution of its definition, and the EBP process. We then determine what is meant by 'evidence' and why hierarchies exist to rank some evidence as stronger than others. Finally, we present current debates and different perspectives on EBP and end by giving some guidance on how you can discuss EBP in your assignments.

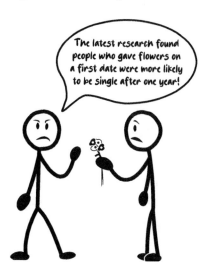

2.2   RELEVANCE: WHY HEALTHCARE PROGRAMMES HAVE EBP MODULES

EBP or research-specific modules are common in all healthcare programmes. Even where there are no dedicated modules, assignment briefs and learning outcomes across several modules will specify that students need to demonstrate their ability to locate, understand, appraise, and apply evidence to various health topics. But why is this the case?

Although the use and role of evidence in practice are not always obvious, think for a moment what practice would look like if it was not informed by research evidence, and was instead based on what had always seemed to work. Do you think we could still advance patient care? Improve patient outcomes? Make the experience of being a service user better? The answer is no. To effectively navigate the evolving healthcare landscape, manage complex illnesses, meet the needs of diverse communities and collaborate within a multidisciplinary team, you must be able to engage with evidence.

In professional terms, EBP is an essential criterion for being a health registrant, as it supports standards of autonomy, accountability, and the maintenance of appropriate knowledge and skills. Being competent to engage with a range of evidence means that we can make informed judgements, as part of a healthcare team. This enables us to offer balanced advice to patients about what interventions may be most effective and what side effects might occur. It means we can work with our practice teams to decide what shift patterns might be safest and what skills are essential for the role. It helps us to weigh up the costs and benefits of a new health facility and how that might meet the needs of a particular community. It should come as no surprise, then, that EBP is embedded in our professional codes, meaning that it is a *requirement* of professional practice to be able to use evidence rather than an optional extra. Box 2.1 gives examples of some regulatory codes of practice and emphasises that joining a professional register means we are agreeing to practice in an evidence-based way.

Box 2.1   Extracts from Professional Codes

The Code (NMC 2018a, p. 9)

6. Always practise in line with the **best available evidence**

To achieve this, you must:

6.1. make sure that any information or advice given is **evidence-based** including information relating to using any health and care products or services

Standards of Proficiency for healthcare professionals (HCPC 2023a–c)

11. assure the quality of their practice
11.1. engage in EBP

11.2. gather and use feedback and information, including qualitative and quantitative data, to evaluate the response of service users to their care

Assistant Practitioner (Health) Occupational Standard (Institute for Apprenticeships and Technical Education 2016)

Knowledge

- **Research** and development in the health and social care sector to inform and improve quality of care
- **Duty 10** Promote an evidence-based approach to providing health and care services, participating in quality improvement and research activity

In personal terms, there are additional benefits from developing EBP skills. Being able to acquire, understand, and apply evidence related to your field of practice can increase your confidence in practice within your team and when interacting with patients. More broadly, being proficient with evidence can encourage personal development and a self-motivated learning mindset that can help you problem-solve and manage challenges in all areas of life. What's not to love about that?

Having said that, we know it can feel like EBP is far removed from real life, conducted and reported by some distant researchers who understand little about the front line of providing care. But often those researchers are health professionals like you, and EBP is a way of bridging the gap between the vast bank of research evidence and the everyday world of practice.

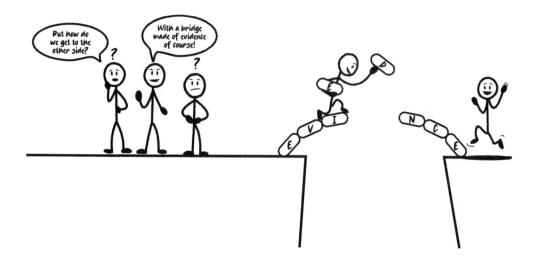

So, your EBP modules and assignments are there to help you personally and professionally to understand the most effective ways of delivering healthcare, and to develop the skills to use evidence to improve your own practice interests.

Assignment Tip

EBP assignments vary considerably in their expected scope and focus, so you should check that you are clear on the assessment brief and learning outcomes for your specific module. For example, while most assignments will require a robust discussion of what EBP is and how it supports good practice, you should clarify how much is expected in terms of the related history, theory, and current debates. Key issues relating to EBP include the following, so check with your tutor if you are unsure:

- The relevance of EBP to healthcare professions
- The historical development of EBP
- The evolving definition of EBP
- The process of EBP and how it works in practice
- Types of evidence and evidence hierarchies
- Debates and criticisms about EBP

2.3 DEVELOPMENT: WHERE DID EBP COME FROM?

EBP is one of the most important developments of the last 50 years for helping health-care professionals to provide safe and effective patient care. It evolved from EBM, a term that was coined in the early 1990s by Gordon Guyatt, although the foundation for the EBM movement was laid many years before (Smith and Rennie 2014).

One of the earliest examples of using an evidence-based approach to inform practice was the investigation of pleural fever following childbirth in the 1800s. Ignaz P. Semmelweis was a Hungarian physician and scientist who noticed that women who were supported by physicians had a higher rate of pleural fever and death than those who were supported by midwives. He investigated and tested possible theories for this

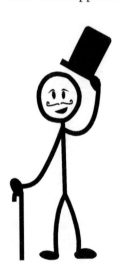

difference in mortality rates and concluded that it was related to the physicians performing autopsies before attending the labouring women (Best and Neuhauser 2004). His findings led to the recommendation that doctors who perform autopsies should wash their hands prior to delivering a baby. Although the recommendation was contested by some, it was implemented, and led to a reduction in maternal deaths (Best and Neuhauser 2004) and sepsis in newborn babies from 18% to 3% (Cwikel 2008).

Another famous figure of the nineteenth century with a commitment to the systematic collection of health data was Florence Nightingale. Nightingale was an accomplished statistician and used her skills during the Crimean war to measure the differences in mortality rates from, for example, wounds and diseases (MacDonald 2001). She was also a pioneer of graphically representing statistical data, using bar charts and pie charts to communicate her findings to the politicians and senior civil servants who could support the changes she wanted to make (McDonald 2001). These early advocates spearheaded the systematic collection and analysis of health data to improve understanding of disease and patient outcomes long before the term EBP evolved (Mackey and Bassendowski 2017).

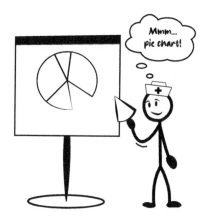

The origins and founding principles of EBP are often attributed to the work of Archie Cochrane in the 1970s. Cochrane was a champion of experimental clinical trials and led the call for physicians only to use treatments that had been shown to be effective through this kind of rigorous investigation. Although controversial at the time, his ideas led to much-needed debate about the fact that medical decision-making was largely based on the clinical experience and knowledge of individual physicians (Mackey and Bassendowski 2017). This meant that there was wide variation in the medical interventions that were offered and uncertainty about which were the safest, most effective, and most cost efficient. To address these issues, Cochrane called for medical interventions to be systematically investigated using research, and for those individual investigations to be collated and reviewed to create a reliable body of evidence that health professionals could use to guide their practice. These collections of research evidence are now generally referred to as 'systematic reviews' and they follow a rigorous process to ensure objectivity and accuracy (Cochrane Collaboration 2023). Cochrane called for the consistent use of randomised controlled trials (RCTs), a specific type of research study, which he argued provided robust evidence on the effectiveness of treatment and led to the writing of his famous book *Effectiveness and Efficiency* (Cochrane 1972).

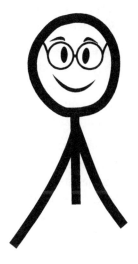

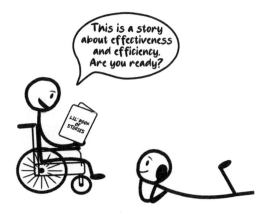

Research Essentials

Research is one source of evidence for EBP. It is characterised by the aim of generating new knowledge through a systematic process of enquiry that involves the collection and analysis of data, related to an explicit research question. There is both primary and secondary research evidence. Find out more about this in Chapter 5.

Primary research has the unique characteristic that new data are collected from participants. The data are collected and then analysed using methods that are appropriate for the research question or aim.

Secondary research collects no new data but instead gathers and analyses existing evidence on a topic to address the review question or aim.

Randomised controlled trials (RCTs) are one type of primary research design. They are highly controlled clinical experiments where people are chosen to receive an intervention, or not, completely at random. This random allocation is key to determining the difference between the results for those who receive an intervention and those who do not. Find out more about RCTs in Chapter 7.

Systematic reviews are rigorous summaries of research evidence, typically of RCT designs, that have been compiled in an objective manner, according to a recognised and documented set of steps. Systematic reviews are a type of secondary research and you can find out more about these in Chapters 4 and 10.

The call for systematic reviews of healthcare interventions led to the creation of the Cochrane Centre, founded in Cochrane's name after his death in 1985. This centre later became the Cochrane Collaboration and is now an important international network providing rigorously appraised evidence to inform healthcare decision-making on a free-to-use website (Cochrane Community 2023).

 Explore It

Have a look at the Cochrane resources to understand their relevance to healthcare.
   First visit the Cochrane website and familiarise yourself with the organisation, its aims, and what it does: www.cochrane.org.
   After this go to the Cochrane Library: www.cochranelibrary.com.
   Note the difference between these sites and consider how the Cochrane Library can help inform decision-making in practice.

2.4   DEFINITIONS: WHAT IS EBP?

The most-cited definition of EBP originates from the work of David Sackett, although it actually relates to EBM. Sackett, a pioneer of clinical epidemiology, is regarded by many as the father of EBM, as he taught medical students that patient care should be informed by scientific evidence rather than tradition or expert opinion (Box 2.2).

Sackett et al.'s (1996) definition reflects the following elements of EBM as it was considered at the time:

- Current best evidence
- Making decisions about patients
- Using clinical expertise alongside research evidence

These demonstrate that up-to-date and high-quality research evidence is central to EBP and suggests that to judge this, research needs to be appraised. Sackett et al.'s (1996) definition also refers to decision-making informed by clinical experience, rather than suggesting that research evidence alone should direct health professionals. Four years later Sackett et al. (2000) updated their definition to:

The integration of best available evidence, clinical expertise and patient preferences and values. (Sackett et al. 2000, p. 1)

 **Checkpoint Activity**   **Aim:** To understand how the definition of EBP has changed.

Instructions: Compare Sackett et al.'s (1996) definition to Sacket et al.'s (2000) definition. What is the same and what is different?

Box 2.2   David Sackett and His Definition of EBP

Evidence-based medicine is the conscientious, explicit, and judicious use of current best evidence in making decisions about the care of individual patients. The practice of evidence-based medicine means integrating individual clinical expertise with the best available external evidence from systematic research. (Sackett et al. 1996 p. 71)

Perhaps you noticed that the definition of EBP has evolved away from making decisions *about* patients to focusing on patient preferences and values, reflecting the shift towards more patient-centred care. The three core components of EBP can now been seen as evidence, expertise, and patients.

EBP is now integral to different fields of healthcare (Satterfield et al. 2009) and its principles are integrated into healthcare policy, driving the development of organisations such as the National Institute for Health and Care Excellence (NICE) and the Scottish Intercollegiate Guidelines Network (SIGN). These organisations act as a bridge between research and practice as they gather a range of evidence, appraise its quality and the strength of its conclusions, and offer guidance for how health professionals might use it.

 Assignment Tip

When using definitions in assignments, do not simply quote someone else. Instead, analyse the definition and make notes about what stands out about it, if it is considered seminal or contemporary, and how it contrasts with other definitions. Remember you are being assessed on your understanding of the topic, so just quoting sources could suggest that you do not understand the concept enough to explain it yourself.

EBP has also become a subject with distinct specialist areas such as evidence-based public health and evidence-based social work (see Box 2.3). Various modifications now exist, with each specialty adapting the original EBM definition to fit the relevant scope of practice (Sattterfield et al. 2009). While these variations can be a little confusing, they demonstrate how integrated the evidence-based approach now is within modern healthcare.

Box 2.3   Derivatives of EBP

Evidence-based public health: 'A public health endeavour in which there is an informed, explicit, and judicious use of evidence that has been derived from any of a variety of science and social science research and evaluation methods' (Rychetnik et al. 2004, p. 538).

Evidence-based nursing: 'An ongoing process by which evidence, nursing theory and the practitioners' clinical expertise are critically evaluated and considered, in conjunction with patient involvement, to provide delivery of optimum nursing care for the individual' (Scott and McSherry 2009, p. 1089).

Evidence-based social work: 'A process designed to forward effective use of professional judgement in integrating information regarding each client's unique characteristics and circumstances, including their preferences and actions, and external research findings' (Gambrill 2003, p. 4).

Evidence-based healthcare: 'A multi-professional approach to using and implementing the best available evidence to ensure the clinically and cost-effective treatment of patients and practice' (Deighan and Boyd 1996, p. 334).

An EBP definition we have found particularly useful is this one from the Joanna Briggs Institute (JBI), an international research organisation based in Australia:

Clinical decision-making that considers the best available evidence; the context in which the care is delivered, client preference and the professional judgment of the health professional (Jordan et al. 2019, p. 58).

This definition has broad appeal for a range of healthcare professions and settings through its use of the term 'client' rather than patient. The retention of 'clinical decision-making' reinforces the idea that EBP cannot prescribe care but instead supports professionals to develop individualised approaches to care. Lastly, it brings the context of care into focus. Whether it is an operating theatre, a home, a clinic, or a community centre, the healthcare setting has a significant bearing on how evidence can be applied, and therefore is a vital part of any contemporary definition.

Overall, the definitions tell us that EBP is not simply using research in practice. EBP is an active process of which *you* are a crucial part. Healthcare professionals exercise their clinical judgement to integrate a range of evidence with patient needs and contextual factors. These elements are captured in various EBP models, which are useful for visualising how they interact (see Figure 2.1).

While the concepts in Figure 2.1 can be considered the core elements of EBP, it's helpful also to identify what kind of contextual factors might come into play, since these may dictate if and how evidence can be applied. Of course, these factors will vary widely depending on the type of healthcare setting, but can be broadly categorised as follows:

- **Ethical and legal considerations:** such as professional codes, ethical principles, and related legislation.
- **Organisational context:** such as formal procedures for changing practice, local policies, and type of culture.
- **Available resources:** such as staffing and costs of implementing an intervention, and equipment available in the setting.

For example, if a treatment was supported by research evidence but was unaffordable for the healthcare organisation, or unwanted by the patient, then it would not be

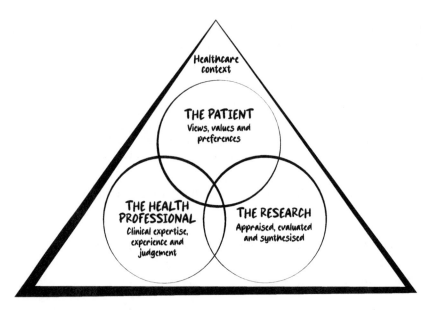

FIGURE 2.1   Basic model of EBP.

feasible or ethical to enforce it and other options would need to be considered. In this scenario, practice is still evidence-based because professional judgement is being used to weigh up the appropriate options given the various considerations. Figure 2.2 provides an advanced model of EBP that includes these additional factors that are important in the application of EBP.

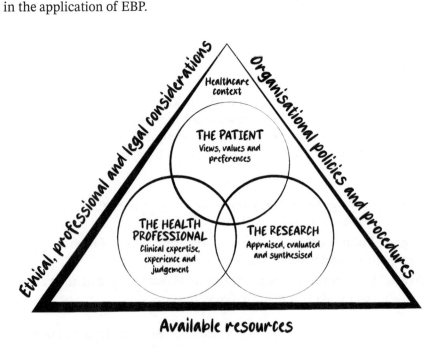

FIGURE 2.2   Advanced model of EBP.

While the definitions and models shown here are useful for explaining the separate components and how they relate, that are not necessarily helpful for illustrating how EBP works in practice. So let us now consider the process of EBP and its different stages that support the use of evidence in healthcare settings.

2.5   PROCESS: HOW DOES EBP WORK?

EBP is described as a problem-solving approach (Melnyk et al. 2010). A problem-solving approach to anything first requires the problem to be defined, after which a solution can be found.

Aim: To reflect on the process of decision-making

Checkpoint Activity

Instructions: Imagine that you want to go on a skiing holiday in France but do not know the best resort, that your washing machine has just broken and you do not know a good appliance repair shop, or that you have had a row with a friend and you cannot decide if you should say sorry. What are the steps you might take to solve these problems? What information would help you to reach a solution?

In a simple problem-solving approach, the following steps help us to reach a solution:

1. **Define:** Before starting to solve the problem, you must understand it. What is it that you are trying to solve? What goal will you achieve through the solution?
2. **Explore:** This is the messy bit! In this step you are collating resources, assimilating information, and getting lost on Google. You are making decisions about which information is more persuasive than others, e.g. the reviews of the resort may have more impact on your decision-making than the photos on the website. You will also be thinking about other factors too, such as the cost and consequences of the possible solutions in front of you.
3. **Choose:** Once you have exhausted the relevant information that informs your decision, you can finally choose a solution. This solution will meet your goal, is within budget, and has the least negative consequences.
4. **Action:** Here is when you take decisive action by implementing the choice you have made in Step 3, and this may require planning. What do you need to execute your decision in a way that will not increase the negative consequences you have assessed in Step 2?
5. **Review:** In this final step you are reflecting on what you did, what worked well, and what did not. You will decide if your choice was the right one, and what you would do if faced with a similar problem in the future.

Now let's compare this simple problem-solving approach to the process of EBP, where Melnyk et al. (2010) and Flemming (2007) both suggest five steps:

1. **Asking** a clinical question: uncertainty from practice is converted into a focused question to trigger the process.
2. **Searching** for the best evidence: the focused question directs a systematic search for relevant research evidence.
3. **Appraising** the evidence: the gathered research is critically evaluated for quality and applicability.
4. **Integrating** the evidence: the gathered research is critically considered alongside the relevant clinical expertise and patient preferences and values.
5. **Evaluating** the outcomes of practice decisions or changes based on the evidence: this might be via a process of self-reflection, audit, or formal research.

These steps can be easily remembered as the 5As: Ask, Acquire, Appraise, Apply, and Assess (Guyatt and Meade 2015).

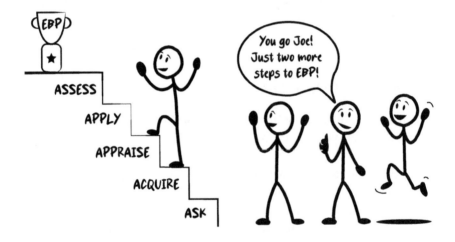

The 5As are often presented in a cyclical format emphasising the iterative, as opposed to linear, nature of the EBP process.

 Assignment Tip

When discussing the process of EBP, do not just describe or list the steps. Make your writing more analytical by, for example, comparing the stages that different authors discuss, applying them within a professional context, or selecting one or two stages for deeper discussion, using a couple of different sources in support.

2.6   HIERARCHIES: WHAT EVIDENCE IS BEST?

We have explained that EBP involves collating and synthesising a range of evidence, but not all evidence is equal. Some types of evidence are stronger and more persuasive in their conclusions than others. Furthermore, depending on the problem being investigated, certain types of evidence may be more applicable than others. So what types of evidence should be considered and how do you know which is most relevant for informing practice?

Let us start by considering what we mean by evidence. Knowing, understanding, and being sure about what is going on are important human needs. It is instinctive to give meaning to life events, to understand how things work and why things happen, and to be able to predict what might happen next. Evidence can be thought of as the things that make us feel sure about what we are doing.

In everyday life our evidence comes from a wide range of sources, all differing in usefulness, value, and accuracy, for example evidence from our experience, from what we have observed, from our cultural beliefs, and from formal education.

We might consider some of this evidence to be more useful than others, perhaps because we feel we can trust it more. This might be because it is something held to be true by our family members, or because it came from someone in authority. This will of course differ from person to person, depending on factors like individual values and cultural backgrounds. Consequently, what is important to me might not be important to you. The same is true in healthcare practice. Some evidence is considered more reliable or relevant than others, and this may differ according to individuals or professional group.

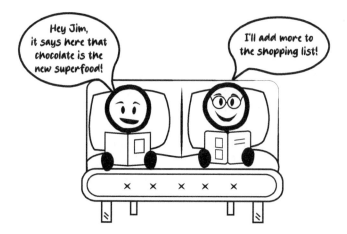

In healthcare there is also a vast amount of evidence available to us. Deciding which is the best quality or most useful for the clinical scenario at hand can be difficult for health professionals. Evidence hierarchies provide a simple guide for deciding which types of evidence may be more reliable than others.

There are many different hierarchies, but the most common form is the pyramid shape, which ranks research designs from the weakest at the bottom to the strongest

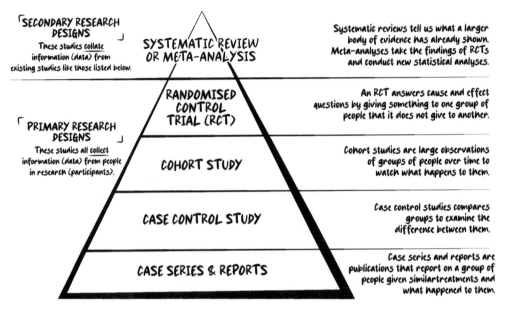

FIGURE 2.3   Traditional hierarchy of evidence explained.

at the top, with strength decided on the potential of the research design to reduce bias and therefore increase the accuracy of the findings. As Figure 2.3 shows, this traditional hierarchy tends to place synthesised collections of evidence (like systematic reviews and meta-analyses) as the strongest form of research evidence and case series/case reports as the weakest.

Hierarchies based on the ability of a research design to control bias have been criticised. RCT designs, for example, are frequently ranked higher than other designs, yet a poorly conducted RCT would not be stronger evidence than a well-conducted observational design like a cohort study (Booth 2010). Therefore, like all models, evidence hierarchies tend to oversimplify a complex set of considerations.

Consequently, some authors have questioned whether evidence hierarchies serve a useful purpose in healthcare (Clark et al. 2018) because they reinforce a narrow view of what valuable and legitimate research is (Holmes et al. 2006). Further to this, hierarchies usually exclude qualitative research designs, which has led to an assumption that qualitative research is not as valuable in healthcare as quantitative research. While it is true that qualitative designs do not focus on reducing bias, they do provide a way of understanding complex human experience that is just as important.

 Research Essentials

Observational research: Non-experimental research.

Cohort study: Research that typically follows a group of people over time to observe what happens to them.

Case–control study: Research that compares those with a disease or other outcome of interest to those without.

Case series/case reports: Clinical description of an individual case of interest, or a series of cases.

Hierarchy: a simple system for ranking items in order of importance or influence.

Meta-analysis: Often used in conjunction with a systematic review to quantitatively synthesise the evidence in the gathered research using statistical analysis to combine the results of multiple studies and generate a more precise estimate of the effect of an intervention or treatment.

Data: a unit of information that, in the context of EBP, relates to information collected from participants to be analysed.

 Assignment Tip

If you are including a discussion of evidence hierarchies in your assignment, try not to simply describe what it is. Apply it to the research you are appraising, to support an evaluation of the research design. Challenge yourself to critically debate how hierarchies can oversimplify the value of different types of evidence, using some additional sources. You could include a more contemporary hierarchy of evidence and why it would be more useful than the traditional version presented in this chapter.

2.7   DEBATE: WHAT ARE THE CRITICISMS OF EBP?

It is important to acknowledge that although EBP is widely embedded within healthcare, there are criticisms and counterarguments you should be aware of. For example, there is concern that EBP creates a regimented or 'recipe' approach to healthcare. It is also argued that EBP prioritises experimental research over other types of evidence, such as qualitative research, clinical expertise, and patient preferences. It is therefore suggested that EBP is not always consistent with individualised patient-centred care (Greenhalgh et al. 2014).

Furthermore, the evidence base itself may misrepresent the truth. The evidence base is often skewed in favour of 'positive results' because studies are easier to publish where the intervention is found to be effective. Moreover, the pharmaceutical industry has been accused of only reporting positive results to skew the weight of evidence in its favour so that it may gain financially (Every-Palmer and Howick 2014). There have even been incidents of research data suppression from clinical trials (Turner et al. 2008), where evidence of unfavourable side effects or harm from new medical products has been hidden from publication.

Evidence can also be misused to suit agendas other than for the direct benefit of patients. This includes cost savings, where organisations may choose to adopt favourable evidence if it reduces care bills and to ignore evidence that might increase costs.

 Explore It

In the UK, the Medicines and Healthcare products Regulatory Agency and the Health Research Authority have advocated for legislation for all clinical trials to register with a national database, so that studies can be monitored for reporting their data in full, and potentially sanctioned if they fail to comply. The Health Research Authority has launched a campaign called *Make it Public* to help ensure that all research is registered and carried out transparently:

`https://www.hra.nhs.uk/planning-and-improving-research/policies-standards-legislation/research-transparency/make-it-public-campaign-group`

EBP has contributed to the production of greater quantities of research evidence, but this is not equal across all health conditions. Some topics, such as new and potentially profitable pharmaceuticals, draw a high degree of research funding and interest. However others, particularly infectious and parasitic diseases that affect poor and marginalised populations disproportionally (Morel 2003), tend to be less supported by research funding and therefore produce less evidence for practice. Greater amounts of evidence also mean that health professionals must have highly developed skills of acquiring, appraising, and applying various types of research evidence to ensure that care is based on all available quality evidence (Greenhalgh et al. 2014).

More recently there have been questions regarding the sustainability of EBP in the light of the evidence required to manage the COVID-19 pandemic (Greenhalgh 2020). The urgent nature of the pandemic and the need to learn quickly about, for example, the efficacy of mask-wearing, coronavirus treatments, and its long-term effects meant that researchers could not lean on traditional 'gold standard' experimental research designs. Instead, they needed to use designs categorised as weaker evidence such as non-randomised and cohort studies. This has generated a fresh debate about what is considered 'suitable' evidence and how EBP can inform whole-population health, rather than having an individual or national-level focus.

This discussion has explained that EBP is a well-established but continually evolving process that can, if health professionals actively engage with its principles and stages, support effective and safe healthcare. We have emphasised that research is just one of a range of types of evidence that might be used, and that professional judgement must be exercised to ensure the evidence aligns with the individual needs of the patient and the specific conditions of the setting. We have also considered the counterarguments to EBP and that, like any movement or approach, negative or unintended consequences must be examined and addressed to maximise the benefits. Now we can explore how to weave all this into your assignment!

2.8   WRITING ABOUT EBP IN YOUR ASSIGNMENT

Let us now consider how you can discuss the fundamental principles and issues of EBP in your assignment. As we have emphasised, you should ensure you are clear about the expectations of your assignment. However, typical requirements may include discussing the historical origins of EBP and its definitions, stages, and relevance to professional practice, and these discussions may form the whole or part of the assignment.

When you are referring to established ideas in your assignments, try to critically discuss different perspectives, and compare them or apply them to the topic your assignment is focused on. Show your awareness of the complexities of EBP, that it is a cyclical and active process rather than a single or linear event. Including the relevance of EBP to professional practice demonstrates that you are able to apply the theory of EBP to your role. Furthermore, by incorporating counterarguments, you can demonstrate a more comprehensive understanding of the process in the real world. See the examples that follow for how some of our students have tackled this.

2.9   ASSIGNMENT EXAMPLES

Example 1: EBP is the process of gathering different types of evidence, one of which is research evidence. Research evidence is characterised by a systematic collection and analysis of data, to investigate a new topic or develop understanding on an existing issue (Jolley 2013). Research is vital to health professionals, to ensure that they are up to date with knowledge of health, illness and treatments and have the capabilities to care for patients safely (Gerrish and Lathlean 2015). The process of evaluating research, known as research appraisal, is essential to make sure that it is reliable and applicable to the particular setting or patient group (Al-Jundi 2017). Nursing Associates must adhere to EBP and develop skills in locating, appraising and using evidence to uphold the requirements of the NMC (2018b).

Example 2: For research to be able to support practice it needs to bridge this 'theory-practice' gap (Jolley 2020). Simply having the knowledge regarding the best evidence is not sufficient, EBP needs to then be implemented into clinical settings (Melnyk and Fineout-Overholt 2019). As part of the Apprenticeship Standards, implementing care in line with current evidence is an essential element of the role of an assistant practitioner (Institute for Apprenticeships and Technical Education 2021).

Example 3: Understanding EBP poses a question as to what is the best available evidence (Ellis 2019). The hierarchy of evidence offers a visual representation of research designs, ranking them from least to most reliable (Ingham-Broomfield 2016). This pyramid only depicts quantitative research methodology (Ellis 2019), with qualitative research criticised as being biased and lacking rigour (Mackieson et al. 2019).

Example 4: Straus et al. (2019) describe EBP as clinical practice shaped by the best clinically relevant and available research, which is influenced by clinical expertise based on experience. It also emphasises the adoption of personalised care and shared decision-making, which is part of the National Health Service (NHS) Long Term Plan (2019). Gerrish and Lathlean (2015) divide EBP into five parts, EBP involves high quality research evidence from primary and secondary studies, professional expertise which is knowledge gained from practical experience, patient preferences regarding treatment, which is weighed against their mental state and health condition. And finally, healthcare resources such as policies and guidelines, these sources of information are taken into consideration when providing evidence-based care (Gerrish and Lathlean 2015).

2.10   END-OF-CHAPTER CHECKPOINT

		Comment/ notes
I can identify three core components of EBP	Yes/no	
I can define evidence-based practice	Yes/no	
I can describe the process of evidence-based practice	Yes/no	
I can discuss hierarchies of evidence and the role of research in advancing patient care	Yes/no	
Now look at the assignment brief or discuss with a module leader and determine which of the following key points should be included in your assignment		
Relevance of EBP to professional practice	Yes/no	
Historical development of EBP	Yes/no	
Contemporary definition of EBP	Yes/no	
The EBP process	Yes/no	
The evidence hierarchy	Yes/no	
Debate of the merits and limitations of EBP	Yes/no	
On a scale of 1–5, how confident do you feel about the content in this chapter?		

2.11 CHAPTER SUMMARY

In this chapter we have introduced the concept of EBP and explained its origins. We have provided a critical discussion of the definitions of EBP and how these evolved from EBM. We have examined the EBP process and the role of hierarchies in assessing the contribution of different types of evidence in decision-making. Finally, we gave you some advice on writing about EBP in assignments and provided some examples. Now we are ready to take a closer look at your assignment task in Chapter 3.

REFERENCES

Al-Jundi, A. (2017). Critical appraisal of clinical research. *Journal of Clinical and Diagnostic Research* 11 (5): JE01–JE05. https://doi.org/10.7860/jcdr/2017/26047.9942.

Best, M. and Neuhauser, D. (2004). Ignaz Semmelweis and the birth of infection control. *BMJ Quality and Safety* 13 (3): 233–234. https://doi.org/10.1136/qshc.2004.010918.

Booth, A. (2010). On hierarchies, malarkeys and anarchies of evidence. *Health Information and Libraries Journal* 27 (1): 84–88. https://doi.org/10.1111/j.1471-1842.2010.00879.x.

Clark, E., Draper, J., and Taylor, R. (2018). Healthcare education research: the case for rethinking hierarchies of evidence. *Journal of Advanced Nursing* 74 (11): 2480–2483. https://doi.org/10.1111/jan.13697.

Cochrane, A.L. (1972). *Effectiveness and Efficiency: Random Reflections on Health Services.* London: Nuffield Provincial Hospitals Trust.

Cochrane Collaboration (2023). About us. https://www.cochrane.org/about-us (accessed 4 December 2023).

Cochrane Community (2023). Archie Cochrane: the name behind Cochrane. https://community.cochrane.org/archie-cochrane-name-behind-cochrane (accessed 4 December 2023).

Cwikel, J. (2008). Lessons from Semmelweis: a social epidemiologic update on safe motherhood. *Social Medicine* 3 (1): 19–35.

Deighan, M. and Boyd, K. (1996). Defining evidence-based health care: a health-care learning strategy? *NT Research* 1 (5): 332–339. https://doi.org/10.1177/136140969600100503.

Ellis, P. (2019). *Evidence-Based Practice in Nursing.* London: Sage.

Every-Palmer, S. and Howick, J. (2014). How evidence-based medicine is failing due to biased trials and selective publication. *Journal of Evaluation in Clinical Practice* 20 (6): 908–914. https://doi.org/10.1111/jep.12147.

Flemming, K. (2007). Asking answerable questions. In: *Evidence-Based Nursing: An Introduction* (ed. N. Cullum, D. Ciliska, B. Haynes, and S. Marks), 18–23. Chichester: Wiley.

Gambrill, E.D. (2003). From the editor. *Journal of Social Work Education* 39 (1): 3–23. https://doi.org/10.1080/10437797.2003.10779115.

Gerrish, K. and Lathlean, J. (2015). *Research Process in Nursing*. Chichester: Wiley Blackwell.

Greenhalgh, T. (2020). Will COVID-19 be evidence-based medicine's nemesis? *PLoS Medicine* 17 (6): e1003266. https://doi.org/10.1371/journal.pmed.1003266.

Greenhalgh, T., Howick, J., and Maskrey, N. (2014). Evidence based medicine: a movement in crisis? *BMJ* 348: g3725. https://doi.org/10.1136/bmj.g3725.

Guyatt, G. and Meade, M.O. (2015). How to use the medical literature – and this book – to improve your patient care. In: *'Users' Guides to the Medical Literature: A Manual for Evidence-Based Clinical Practice*, 3e (ed. G. Guyatt, D. Rennie, M.O. Meade, and D.J. Cook). New York: McGraw-Hill https://jamaevidence.mhmedical.com/content.aspx?bookid=847&sectionid=69030730 (accessed 4 December 2023).

Health & Care Professions Council (HCPC) (2023a). Standards of Proficiency: Occupational Therapists. https://www.hcpc-uk.org/standards/standards-of-proficiency/occupational-therapists (accessed 4 December 2023).

Health & Care Professions Council (HCPC) (2023b). Standards of Proficiency: Operating Department Practitioners. https://www.hcpc-uk.org/standards/standards-of-proficiency/operating-department-practitioners (accessed 4 December 2023).

Health & Care Professions Council (HCPC) (2023c). Standards of Proficiency: Radiographers. https://www.hcpc-uk.org/standards/standards-of-proficiency/radiographers (accessed 4 December 2023).

Holmes, D., Murray, S.J., Perron, A., and Rail, G. (2006). Deconstructing the evidence-based discourse in health sciences: truth, power and fascism. *International Journal of Evidence-Based Healthcare* 4 (3): 180–186. https://doi.org/10.1111/j.1479-6988.2006.00041.x.

Ingham-Broomfield, R. (2016). A nurses' guide to the hierarchy of research designs and evidence. *Australian Journal of Advanced Nursing* 33 (3): 38–43.

Institute for Apprenticeships and Technical Education (2016). Assistant practitioner (health) occupational standard. https://www.instituteforapprenticeships.org/apprenticeship-standards/healthcare-assistant-practitioner?view=standard (accessed 4 December 2023).

Institute for Apprenticeships and Technical Education (2021). Assistant practitioner (health). https://www.instituteforapprenticeships.org/apprenticeship-standards/assistant-practitioner-health-v1-1 (accessed 4 December 2023).

Jolley, J. (2013). *Introducing Research and Evidence-Based Practice for Nursing and Healthcare Professionals*. Abingdon: Routledge.

Jolley, J. (2020). *Introducing Research and Evidence-Based Practice for Nursing and Healthcare Professionals*. London: Routledge.

Jordan, Z., Lockwood, C., Munn, Z., and Aromataris, E. (2019). The updated Joanna Briggs Institute Model of Evidence-Based Healthcare. *JBI Evidence Implementation* 17 (1): 58. https://doi.org/10.1097/XEB.0000000000000155.

Mackey, A. and Bassendowski, S. (2017). The history of evidence-based practice in nursing education and practice. *Journal of Professional Nursing* 33 (1): 51–55. https://doi.org/10.1016/j.profnurs.2016.05.009.

Mackieson, P., Shlonsky, A., and Connolly, M. (2019). Increasing rigor and reducing bias in qualitative research: a document analysis of parliamentary debates using applied thematic analysis. *Qualitative Social Work* 18 (6): 965–980.

McDonald, L. (2001). Florence Nightingale and the early origins of evidence-based nursing. *Evidence-Based Nursing* 4 (3): 68–69. https://doi.org/10.1136/ebn.4.3.68.

Melnyk, B.M. and Fineout-Overholt, E. (2019). *Evidence-Based Practice in Nursing & Healthcare: A Guide to Best Practice*. Philadelphia: Wolters Kluwer.

Melnyk, B.M., Finehout-Overholt, E., Stillwell, S.B., and Williamson, K.B. (2010). Evidence-based practice: step by step: the seven steps of evidence-based practice. *American Journal of Nursing* 110 (1): 51–53. https://doi.org/10.1097/01.NAJ.0000366056.06605.d2.

Morel, C.M. (2003). Neglected diseases: under-funded research and inadequate health interventions. *EMBO Reports* 4 (Suppl 1): S35–S38. https://doi.org/10.1038/sj.embor.embor851.

National Health Service (NHS) (2019). NHS Long Term Plan. https://www.longtermplan.nhs.uk (accessed 4 December 2023).

Nursing and Midwifery Council (NMC) (2018a). The Code: Professional standards of practice and behaviour for nurses, midwives and nursing associates. www.nmc.org.uk/standards/code (accessed 4 December 2023).

Nursing and Midwifery Council (NMC) (2018b). Standards for nursing associates. https://www.nmc.org.uk/standards/standards-for-nursing-associates (accessed 4 December 2023).

Rychetnik, L., Hawe, P., Waters, E. et al. (2004). A glossary for evidence based public health. *Journal of Epidemiology and Community Health* 58 (7): 538–545. https://doi.org/10.1136/jech.2003.011585.

Sackett, D.L., Rosenberg, W.M.C., Gray, J.A.M. et al. (1996). Evidence based medicine: what it is and what it isn't. *BMJ (Clinical Research ed.)* 312 (7023): 71–72. https://doi.org/10.1136/bmj.312.7023.71.

Sackett, D.L., Straus, S.E., Richardson, W.S. et al. (2000). *Evidence-Based Medicine: How to Practice and Teach EBM*, 2e. New York: Churchill Livingstone.

Satterfield, J.M., Spring, B., Brownson, R.C. et al. (2009). Toward a transdisciplinary model of evidence-based practice. *Milbank Quarterly* 87 (2): 368–390. https://doi.org/10.1111/j.1468-0009.2009.00561.x.

Scott, K. and McSherry, R. (2009). Evidence-based nursing: clarifying the concepts for nurses in practice. *Journal of Clinical Nursing* 18 (8): 1085–1095. https://doi.org/10.1111/j.1365-2702.2008.02588.x.

Smith, R. and Rennie, D. (2014). Evidence-based medicine – an oral history. *JAMA* 311 (4): 365–367. https://doi.org/10.1001/jama.2013.286182.

Straus, S.E., Glasziou, P., Richardson, W.S., and Haynes, R.B. (2019). *Evidence-based Medicine: How to Practice and Teach EBM*. Edinburgh: Elsevier.

Turner, E.H., Matthews, A.M., Linardatos, E. et al. (2008). Selective publication of antidepressant trials and its influence on apparent efficacy. *New England Journal of Medicine* 358 (3): 252–260. https://doi.org/10.1056/NEJMsa065779.

CHAPTER 3

The Task at Hand

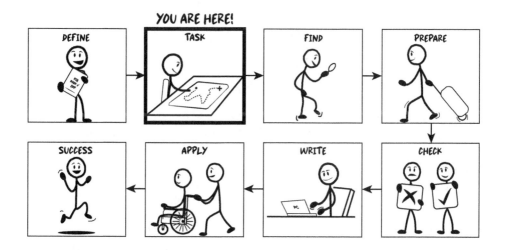

FIVE THINGS TO LEARN FROM THIS CHAPTER

1. Knowing the learning outcomes and following assessment module guidelines are key to a successful assignment.
2. The EBP process is often adapted for an assignment to make it more feasible within the time frame. So you need to have clarity on what stage(s) need to be completed.

Critical Appraisal Skills for Healthcare Students: A Practical Guide to Writing Evidence-based Practice Assignments, First Edition. Charlotte J. Whiffin, Donna Barnes, and Lorraine Henshaw.
© 2024 John Wiley & Sons Ltd. Published 2024 by John Wiley & Sons Ltd.

3. If you are allowed to choose your own topic area, select a subject that you are passionate about and that concerns a relevant patient population.

4. A question is required to lead the EBP process. Good questions can be developed using frameworks such as PICO, PICOT, PEO, PIO, SPIDER, and SPICE.

5. Structured questions are important for focused searching and appropriate selection of literature.

FIVE MINUTES WITH JACK, OCCUPATIONAL THERAPY STUDENT

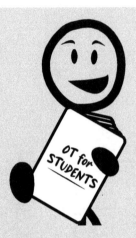

How did you feel at the start of the module?
To begin with I was nervous and apprehensive, I did not feel I'd ever have the confidence to state if a piece of research wasn't reliable or that I would be able to spot any areas of improvement with the research. You assume because it's been published it will be a credible piece of evidence.

Did anything help you overcome these difficulties?
I wrote a plan of what I wanted to include in each section of my assignment. This enabled me to keep on track of what information needed to go into the correct section.

How did you start writing your assignment?
Using headings to ensure each learning outcome was being addressed; these headings can be deleted at a later date if necessary.

What advice would you give to others starting an EBP module?
Do not let a preconceived opinion formed by negative feedback from other students affect your research journey.
Read as much as you can, as you may come across new terms that may not have been covered within the units and could get you extra marks.

> Choose a study that you are interested in and a methodology that aligns with your preference. Start writing as early as you can and bring forward your deadline in case of any last-minute panics!
> Try not to get overwhelmed, it will all make sense in the end. If you are unsure of anything ask your module tutor.

3.1   INTRODUCTION

In this chapter we consider the task at hand. While the 'task' will differ for different students, there are some commonalities when it comes to writing assignments, especially those that require completion of a critical appraisal activity. Therefore, this chapter has lots of checkpoints and activities to complete and we will share our collective experience of marking student assignments to help guide you towards a successful submission. That said, you need to understand the learning outcomes, academic level, and marking criteria for the assignment you are writing and apply the principles described in this chapter. You should also engage fully with your module tutors and absorb the advice they provide.

3.2   THE IMPORTANCE OF LEARNING OUTCOMES

You will not pass an assignment if you have not met the learning outcomes, no matter how well you have written the assignment! Therefore, the learning outcomes, and any additional assessment guidance, provide a framework for you to write your assignment. However, learning outcomes can be quite broad, so there are often different ways these can be interpreted or achieved. This is when additional assignment guidance can be helpful, which may be in written or verbal form and should be provided by the module team. Armed with this information you will have the scaffolding you need to write the assignment in a style that suits your profession, your experience, and your emerging confidence.

3.3   HOW TO FOLLOW THE EBP PROCESS FOR AN ASSIGNMENT

Following a comprehensive EBP process from start to end within the confines of an academic assignment is very difficult, unless that assignment is an extended piece of work like a dissertation. Therefore, in an EBP or research module you may be asked to follow a stage, or stages, in a way that is more feasible within a shortened time frame. Table 3.1 lists several ways the EBP process can be shortened for an academic assignment.

TABLE 3.1   Ways to engage in EBP for a summative assignment.

EBP assignment shortcut	Pros	Cons
Topic pre-determined by module team.	Keeps you focused so you are quicker to start the assignment.	Low level of control – you may not be interested in the topics chosen so you may disengage more easily.
Papers for appraisal are set by the module team.	Saves time as you do not have to locate the papers yourself Reduces your frustration with database searching. You will definitely have appropriate papers to critique The module team will know how to guide your appraisal.	Low level of control – you may not be interested in the topics chosen so you may disengage more easily. You do not learn database searching skills. Appraisal can be harder if the topic is not one of interest to you.
Limited number of papers for review.	Makes the assignment feasible given the time constraint.	Limits your understanding of the wider evidence base and therefore its application to practice.
Tools to facilitate appraisal chosen by the module team.	Saves you time, as you know the tool is appropriate for your assignment and you do not need to look at different tools.	Reduced exposure to different ways to appraise research. You may not like the tool chosen by the module team.

Table 3.1 also illustrates just some of the different ways an EBP assignment can be approached and should demonstrate to you the importance of clarifying exactly what it is you must do to pass. Clarity on this point is essential. A particularly common way in which an EBP assignment can differ from a fully operationalised EBP task is by limiting the number of papers you are expected to critically appraise. In a formal EBP task the aim is to source all the relevant evidence that answers the clinical question set at the start of the process. In an extended assignment, like a dissertation, you may need to limit this to 10–15 individual research papers so the review can be completed within the year that is typical for these sorts of modules. However, for a research or EBP module you may only be asked to review a more limited evidence base (perhaps just one or two papers), so you need to be very clear from the outset how many papers you are required to review.

Finally, if you are allowed to select your own papers for review, you may also want to check what type of evidence you need to appraise for your assignment. Chapter 4 looks more closely at the different types of evidence you will find; however, at this stage just knowing whether there are specific requirements for the module is helpful. For example, you may be directed to primary research only, or to a particular research design like a randomised controlled trial.

Assignment Tip

There is a lot of evidence in the evidence base, so be clear from the outset how many papers you need to appraise and what type of evidence is appropriate for your assignment and what is not. If you are allowed to select your own papers, you should explain in your assignment why certain papers have been chosen so your reader can understand your thinking.

Complete the following checklist to ensure you are clear on the assignment requirements.

	Yes	No	Comments
I can choose my own topic			
I need to conduct a database search			
I can choose my own papers			
I know how many papers I must appraise			How many?
I know what types of research papers I must choose			Type of research paper required:
I can choose the critical appraisal tool			If no, the appraisal tool to be used is:
I know the learning outcomes for the module			Learning outcomes are located in:
I have been given verbal and/or written guidelines on how to achieve the learning outcomes			
I understand what I need to do			If no, book in to see your module leader

3.4   CHOOSING A TOPIC

If you are allowed to pick your own topic, this provides a great opportunity to explore the evidence base on an area of practice you feel passionate about. Reading a research paper can be quite a challenging activity because they can be long, written in a style that does not engage you, written using words you are unfamiliar with, and employing methods you do not understand. However, if the paper reports on a subject relevant to your practice or patient group, something you feel passionate about, this will keep you more focused on the task at hand and will help you to reflect on the relevance of the findings to this population. If you are allowed to choose your topic area, reflecting on previous clinical placements is a good starting point for generating areas of interest. Completing the following checkpoint activity will help you to identify a subject of interest.

Aim: To identify a subject of interest for your EBP assignment.

Checkpoint Activity

Instructions: Reflect on your clinical placements or past clinical experiences. Make a list of the patients, conditions, diseases, or treatments that really interested you. List them, then decide which is a possible contender for your assignment.

1.

2.

3.

4.

My potential area of interest is: ....

Now you have a topic of interest, it is useful to identify some key facts about what and who this topic is about. These key facts can be used in the introduction to the assignment and will tell the reader why this topic is important in healthcare. Complete the next checkpoint activity for your identified area of interest.

Aim: To identify key facts.

Checkpoint Activity

Instructions: Answer the following questions. Don't forget to make a note of any references!

1. What is the most cited definition for this subject?
2. How many people does this affect annually?
3. Who does this affect the most?

Once you have a subject area in mind, you need to dig a little more deeply into a specific topic that warrants further attention. Let's consider a broad area of interest like cancer. You need to identify something of particular interest within this subject area. This 'thing', or phenomenon, of interest can be located anywhere from interventions and treatments to subjective experiences of patients or healthcare staff.

Research Essentials

Phenomenon: Researchers often use the term phenomenon or phenomena to describe the event, situation, or circumstances they wish to investigate.

At this stage there may be many different possible phenomena of interest and it is useful to write all these down and keep a track of your thinking. Depending on what experiences you have been exposed to and/or are interested in identifying, the phenomena of interest will either be relatively straightforward or pose a problem because there are too many, or too few. Using the prompts in the next checkpoint activity will help you identify some potential phenomena of interest.

 Aim: To identify a phenomenon of interest relevant to your professional practice.

Instructions: Draw a mind map and place your topic area in the middle. Now add the answers to the following questions:

- What conditions, problems, or interventions are you interested in?
- What do not you understand about this topic area?
- What areas of care could be improved?
- What issues are most relevant to your profession?
- What would you like to know more about?

From these answers, which interests you the most? Place a circle around it – this will be your chosen phenomenon. We have given you an example here. You can do this activity as many times as you like until you identify an area you wish to investigate.

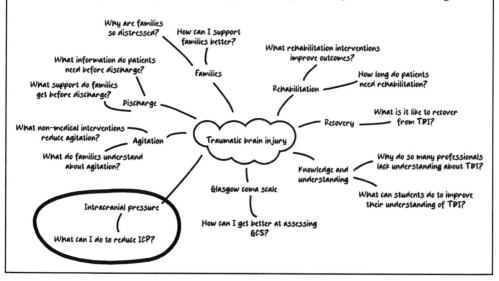

If you do not have a clear topic in mind, you can get a bit overwhelmed and spend too long in this early exploration phase. While it is ideal to choose something you are passionate about and engaged in, remember to be pragmatic too: choose something that is feasible in the time frame and that will help you achieve the learning outcomes for your module. Time is of the essence when writing an assignment, so navigating through the process of identifying a topic is a key milestone that needs to be reached early on. The next checkpoint will get you to delve a little deeper into your phenomenon of interest.

 Checkpoint Activity

Aim: To describe key points.

Instructions: It is now time to identify some key points about the phenomenon of interest. This time, instead of stating the 'what' and the 'who', you need to provide some background information about why this is an important subject area in healthcare and why it is important to your profession. Answer the following questions, and do not forget your references:

1. Why is this an important issue in healthcare?
2. Why is this subject relevant to your professional practice?
3. How would an investigation of this problem improve practice?

Assignment Tip

Assignments commonly start with an introduction to the subject and a statement about why this is an important subject area for professional practice. You can now use the answers from the previous checkpoints to write a short paragraph about the subject. An example is provided here.

Answers from first checkpoint:
(i) Dementia is defined as a general term of the loss of cognitive functioning that interferes with the person's everyday life (CDC 2019). According to the World Health Organization (2023) more than 55 million people have dementia. (ii) Dementia most commonly affects older people with women more disproportionately affected than men.

Answers from second checkpoint:
(i) Dementia rates are rising given our ageing population (Alzheimer's Association 2020). There is no cure for dementia, which means people are living with multiple cognitive deficits and a gradual decline in their level of functioning (Sandilyan and Dening 2015). (ii) Patients with dementia are commonly admitted to acute healthcare settings and this often exacerbates their confusion, causing them and their families distress. (iii) An investigation into an effective way to calm patients with dementia, without using medication, would improve the experience of patients and families when admitted to hospital.

3.5 TURNING A TOPIC INTO A QUESTION

You should now have a reasonable idea of what you want to investigate. However, there may be some benefit in refining this even further in order to help you develop a leading question that marks the start of the EBP process. You many therefore need to think about whether there are any groups you want to focus on, where they are located, what age/sex they are, and perhaps if there are any geographical restrictions. An example of this refining process is provided in the next activity.

 Checkpoint Activity

Aim: To refine your phenomenon of interest.

Instructions: Read the questions and their answers in the following table and then add your answers in the final column.

	Example	Your answers
My topic of interest is:	Cancer	
The phenomenon of interest is:	Organ donation preferences	
The specific people I am most interested in are:	Palliative care patients	
The setting I am considering is:	Acute hospitals	
The people are usually aged:	Over 60	
The sex I am most interested in is:	Female	
The question is most relevant to people in:	UK	

You can see in the example provided that the topic has been refined to 'organ donation preferences of female adult palliative cancer patients in acute hospitals in the UK'. This is a far more focused subject area that can be turned into a question by adding a verb at the start and a question mark at the end:

> **What** *are the organ donation preferences of female palliative cancer patients, over the age of 60, in acute hospitals in the UK?*

Now complete the next checkpoint activity to turn your phenomenon of interest into a question.

Aim: To turn your phenomenon of interest into a question.

Instructions: Use your learning from this chapter and the answers to the questions in the checkpoint activities to identify a question using a verb at the start and a question mark at the end.

My question is: _____

_____

_____

3.6   HOW TO DEVELOP A 'GOOD' QUESTION

Having reached this stage, you should be starting to feel confident that you know what it is you want to achieve and what question you want to answer. However, in the context of EBP questions it is important to set a 'good' question. By a 'good' question we mean one that is focused around the key concepts of interest. These key concepts will guide you later in the search and selection of appropriate evidence, as described in Chapter 4.

Assignment Tip

Your specific assignment may not require you to develop your own searchable question, but it may still be important to demonstrate that you understand the principles of developing a good question and the relevance of this to EBP. Consider discussing the role that question development plays in the EBP process and the facets that contribute to a robust leading question.

For healthcare questions the 'PICO' framework works well (Beecroft et al. 2015). This acronym stands for 'Population, Intervention, Comparison, Outcome' and developed originally from quantitative studies of interventions like clinical trials. In these studies, there is always a *population* of interest, an *intervention* that is being tested, a *control* or *comparison* group and then an *outcome* that is measured to understand whether the intervention was more successful in the intervention or comparison group. This mnemonic 'is a staple of EBP pedagogy' (Schiavenato and Chu 2021).

Here is an example of how these components come together in a question:

Are healthcare staff (population) / who attend a resilience training programme (intervention) / more satisfied with their work (outcome) / than healthcare staff who do not (comparison)?

Time is often added to PICO making it PICOT, which may or may not be relevant to your question, for example one week/month post intervention. However, there are lots of other ways in which a well-defined question can be constructed. These are listed in Table 3.2 with examples. Note that when writing a question you do not need to write each concept in a particular order – they can be moved around to ensure the question is easy to understand and as succinct as possible.

Our experience of helping students to frame their questions using such acronyms is very mixed. Some students find it easy to identify their concepts of interest. Others really struggle to force their area of interest into a framework, often resulting in a question that does not make sense or misrepresents what it is the student wants to achieve. Therefore, we offer an alternative to these acronyms that focuses on the concepts of interest (two examples are provided in Table 3.3). However, using unstructured questions can mean your question is not focused enough, so be careful not to simply take an easy option here only to make mistakes later in your database searches and choice of papers.

TABLE 3.2   EBP question frameworks.

Question type	Example
PICO Population, intervention, comparison, outcome	Is a weight management programme (intervention) for pregnant women (population) more effective for weight loss (outcome) than exercise alone (comparison)?
PICOT Population, intervention, comparison, outcome, time	Are nasal decongestants (intervention) more effective than paracetamol (comparison) at reducing nasal congestion (outcomes) for adults with a common cold (population) within the first four hours of administration (time)?
PIO Population, intervention/ issue, outcome	Are students (population) who access student support (intervention) more satisfied with their university course (outcome)?
PEO Population, exposure, outcome	How do diagnostic radiographers (population) live and work with back pain (outcome) that they attribute to the manual handling practices within their department (exposure)?
SPICE Setting, perspective/ population, intervention, comparison, evaluation	In nursing homes (setting), do therapy dolls (intervention) as opposed to no therapy dolls (comparison), reduce anxiety (evaluation) in patients with dementia (population)?
SPIDER Sample, phenomenon of interest, design, evaluation, research type	How do new parents (sample) describe (evaluation) their qualitative (research type) experience of their infants' failure to thrive (phenomenon of interest) in unstructured interviews (design)?

TABLE 3.3   Examples of unstructured questions.

Unstructured	What does patient centre care (concept 1) mean to radiography (concept 2) students (concept 3)?
	Do patients (concept 1) understand (concept 2) the role of occupational therapists (concept 3)?

3.7 BENEFITS OF A GOOD QUESTION

The main benefit of a focused question is that it provides clarity regarding the task at hand. This question becomes a firm anchor for what you need to achieve in your assignment. Furthermore, if you have a well-structured question this will enable you to conduct a focused search for relevant evidence (see Chapter 4). Without a good question you risk the integrity of all the subsequent stages in the EBP process, your assignment will lack a coherent narrative, and your practice implications will be weaker.

Most often question development is an iterative process that will take more than one attempt to get right. Therefore, you may have to work through the activities in this chapter several times as you change your mind, or you realise that it isn't possible to answer the question you initially set for your assignment. To help in this initial phase of question development, you may want to spend some time searching for possible ideas on the internet, speaking with friends and colleagues, and talking with patients and families following healthcare events.

 Research Essentials

Iterative: Iterative is a term used in research to describe a non-linear process. In such a process the research may take several steps back before being able to move forward, or the process may be repeated several times until an outcome is reached.

Now complete the next checkpoint activity to see if you can use an EBP question framework and improve the question you identified earlier in the chapter.

Aim: To construct a 'good' question.

Instructions: Returning to the question you developed earlier in this chapter, rewrite it using one of the frameworks identified in Table 3.2. Identify each of the concepts within the question, e.g. PIO – Are students (population) who access student support (intervention) more satisfied with their university course (outcome)?

Chosen framework (e.g. PIO, PICO):

Your question:_____

_____

If a framework is not working for you, try to write the question using an unstructured approach like those in Table 3.3. However, remember still to identify each core concept, e.g. What does patient-centred care (concept 1) mean to radiography (concept 2) students (concept 3)?

Your question:_____

_____

You should now have a good question to lead the EBP process and understand the task before you.

3.8   WRITING ABOUT EBP QUESTIONS IN YOUR ASSIGNMENT

First establish if your assignment requires you to discuss the role of a good clinical question in EBP and, if so, to what extent. As a minimum, show that you know how a well-developed question fits within the overall EBP process, and the key elements of a good question. Aim to discuss this rather than making statements by bringing in different perspectives and noting if they clash. If it's appropriate to your assignment, try to apply the issue of a good question to your topic. See the following student examples for how you might tackle this. The second example is from an assignment that required the student to undertake a literature review and develop their own question. Although this may be more typical of a level 6 dissertation, it shows how question frameworks can be used and how EBP knowledge can be put into practice.

3.9   ASSIGNMENT EXAMPLES

Example 1: Search questions can be refined with the help of the 'Patient/Problem/ Population, Intervention, Comparison, Outcome' (PICO) framework to identify key concepts and develop the answerable research question (De Brún 2013).

Example 2: Aveyard and Sharp (2017) suggest using question frameworks such as Population, Intervention, Comparison, Outcome and Time (PICOT) and Sample, Phenomena of Interest, Design, Evaluation and Research (SPIDER) to assist in developing the research question. Methley et al. (2014) argue that the PICOT tool targets several search terms not relevant to qualitative research, such as control group and intervention. Cooke et al. (2012) developed the SPIDER tool to identify qualitative articles further whilst removing irrelevant categories such as the comparison aspect of the PICOT tool (Aveyard and Sharp 2017). The SPIDER tool was appropriate for developing the question for this review, as it enabled a specific focus on a male population and targeting of studies that explored lived experience of this phenomenon. *The review questions was: 'What is the impact pregnancy loss has on males, from their perspective?'*

3.10   END-OF-CHAPTER CHECKPOINT

		Comment/notes
I know the learning outcomes for the module assignment	Yes/no	
I understand how to achieve the learning outcomes	Yes/no	

		Comment/notes
I know the question I want to answer through this assignment	Yes/no	
I know how to use question frameworks like PICO, SPICE and SPIDER	Yes/no	
My leading question is:		
I am interested in the answer to my leading question	Yes/no	If no, you may want to reconsider your question.

On a scale of 1–5, how confident do you feel about the content in this chapter?

3.11   CHAPTER SUMMARY

In this chapter we considered the 'task at hand' – what it is that you have to do for your assignment. It is unfortunate that every year students do not pass modules simply because they have misunderstood what was required of them. By engaging with this chapter you will have clarified the assignment brief, learning outcomes and what topic and question you wish to investigate. Now you will use this question to formulate a robust search strategy in Chapter 4.

REFERENCES

Alzheimer's Association (2020). 2020 Alzheimer's disease facts and figures. *Alzheimer's & Dementia* 16 (3): 391–460.

Aveyard, H. and Sharp, P. (2017). *A Beginner's Guide to Evidence-based Practice in Health and Social Care*, 3e. London: Open University Press.

Beecroft, C., Booth, A., and Rees, A. (2015). Finding the evidence. In: *The Research Process in Nursing*, 7e (ed. K. Gerrish and J. Lathlean), 89–104. Oxford Wiley Blackwell.

Centers for Disease Control and Prevention (2019). Alzheimer's disease and healthy aging. https://www.cdc.gov/aging/dementia/index.html (accessed 4 December 2023).

Cooke, A., Smith, D., and Booth, A. (2012). Beyond PICO: the SPIDER tool for qualitative evidence synthesis. *Qualitative Health Research* 22 (10): 1435–1443. https://doi.org/10.1177/1049732312452938.

De Brún, C. (2013). Useful databases. The Information Standard, November. https://www.england.nhs.uk/tis/wp-content/uploads/sites/17/2014/09/tis-evidence-wrkshp-caroline-de-brun.pdf (accessed 4 December 2023).

Methley, A.M., Campbell, S., Chew-Graham, C. et al. (2014). PICO, PICOS and SPIDER: a comparison study of specificity and sensitivity in three search tools for qualitative systematic reviews. *BMC Health Services Research* 21 (14): 579. https://doi.org/10.1186/s12913-014-0579-0.

Sandilyan, M.B. and Dening, T. (2015). Diagnosis of dementia. *Nursing Standard* 29 (43): 36–41. https://doi.org/10.7748/ns.29.43.36.e9441.

Schiavenato, M. and Chu, F. (2021). PICO: what it is and what it is not. *Nurse Education in Practice* 56: 103194. https://doi.org/10.1016/j.nepr.2021.103194.

World Health Organization. (2023). Fact sheets of dementia. Available from: https://www.who.int/news-room/fact-sheets/detail/dementia (accessed 21 January 2024).

CHAPTER 4

Locating and Identifying Research

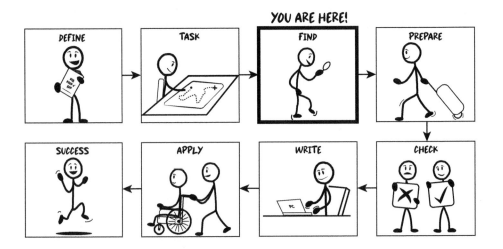

FIVE THINGS TO LEARN FROM THIS CHAPTER

1. Systematic searching is a specific approach to retrieving evidence to answer EBP questions.
2. Systematic searching is the only way to ensure literature retrieval is comprehensive and objective.

Critical Appraisal Skills for Healthcare Students: A Practical Guide to Writing Evidence-based Practice Assignments, First Edition. Charlotte J. Whiffin, Donna Barnes, and Lorraine Henshaw.
© 2024 John Wiley & Sons Ltd. Published 2024 by John Wiley & Sons Ltd.

3. Peer-reviewed research published in healthcare journals can be found by searching healthcare databases.

4. Expect to spend a lot of time developing a robust search method that can be applied in different databases.

5. Your account of your search methods should be detailed enough that someone else could locate the same papers.

FIVE MINUTES WITH DAVID, NURSING ASSOCIATE STUDENT

What search did you have to do for your module?
I already had an interest in my subject area due to a placement I attended and experienced firsthand. I decided to research this area more for my assessment. The search I had to do was to find relevant articles in this field to try and answer a specific research question. I did have to learn more about the methodology for the search to make sure this was accurate and that I found the right articles. I read a lot of books to help with my under-standing, finding glossaries for words I was unsure of.

Did you find it easy to search for articles?
Although I did have some understanding of how to search for arti-cles, I also attended extra sessions at the library. This was face to face and I attended two online sessions during year 2 as this was during COVID-19. This really helped and when I completed the research module I found searching for articles much easier.

If you had to do the same search again, would you do anything differently?
In the beginning, I was worrying a lot about how to get things started or if the articles I had found were good enough. I did eventually seek help from my tutor, who put my mind at rest and went through everything with me. In the end I knew I had the understanding and knowledge of the search methodology when I was doing it and I understood what was needed. What I wish is that I had more of an understanding of the tools available to screen, filter, and eliminate the articles that I did not need. I had to research around those, which at the time felt like extra work, as I do not remember discussing those during lectures, etc., it was mainly through the library sessions I completed.

What advice would you give another student about to embark on a database search?
Seek help if you are not sure, whether it be from the tutors or the librarians. Read around the areas you are not clear about, read to understand the words and what is being asked of you. There are also some useful guides on the database help pages that can help.

4.1   INTRODUCTION

This chapter will expand on what is needed to search for evidence in a formal way, known as 'systematic searching'. The chapter is particularly useful for those who need to conduct a literature search as part of their EBP assignment. Although not all EBP assignments will require students to source their own studies (for example, module tutors may have pre-sourced these for you), the principles laid out in this chapter are fundamental to EBP and as such healthcare professionals should be proficient in these skills.

It is natural to think that locating and identifying research should be easy. After all, we use search engines all the time trying to locate anything from the nearest supermarket to the best recipe for chocolate cake. Many people have grown up with the internet so electronic searching is part of their DNA. Even without this experience, we all now expect instant access to the best journals and most up-to-date research with little effort. While online searching, e-journals and open access bring enormous benefit, they have also made us a little lazy. We have fallen into bad habits like limiting searching to full text and ignoring subject-specific databases in favour of search engines like Google and Google Scholar. While these have their place in searching, this chapter is focused on reorientating you to the systematic requirements of literature retrieval as would be expected within the EBP process. So here is a slight warning: be prepared to *unlearn* some of your bad habits and go the long way around. Then if you choose to cut a corner in the future, you will know what corner you have cut and understand the implications of that for your retrieval of literature.

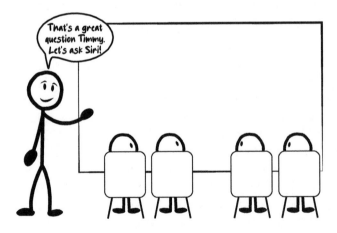

4.2   HOW MUCH TIME DO YOU HAVE?

The first question you should ask is how much time you have to conduct your search. If you only have a few minutes, you cannot conduct a thorough search of the evidence base (De Brún and Pearce-Smith 2014). To do this properly you need to set aside a few hours at least and be prepared for several searching sessions before you get to what you need. So the bottom line is: do not expect searching properly to be a quick process! Rather than squeeze it into five minutes, give searching the time it deserves.

4.3   WHY ARE YOU SEARCHING FOR LITERATURE?

Before you start searching for literature, you need to be clear on the purpose and intended outcome of this process. Literature retrieval for an assignment is quite different to the process expected in a literature review, for example. Literature reviews that require a systematic approach to literature retrieval need to have clear and detailed methods for how the search is conducted. The search principles and techniques outlined here are important to know and become proficient in. However, when writing a general assignment, you do not normally need to demonstrate that you have sourced the leading evidence in the field and how you found it. In contrast, if you are writing an assignment on the EBP process that requires you to conduct a systematic search, then your methods of literature retrieval will be assessed. In this case, a systematic search should be comprehensive and repeatable (Harari et al. 2020). The subsequent sections of this chapter will help you to develop a clear search strategy that fits the purpose of your assignment.

 Research Essentials

Literature review: 'The comprehensive study and interpretation of literature that address a specific question' (Aveyard 2019).

Systematic searching: 'the process of locating the literature which answers a specific question' (Davis 2016).

Repeatability is a really important aspect of literature reviews, as others need to be able to repeat your search and check your sources if they need to.

In systematic searching the search is *so* important that if you get it wrong, you risk undermining the whole project. As a result, you need to commit the time and effort required for this process. You will need to develop a search strategy that will ensure you look for research in the correct way and such that others would be able to follow your steps.

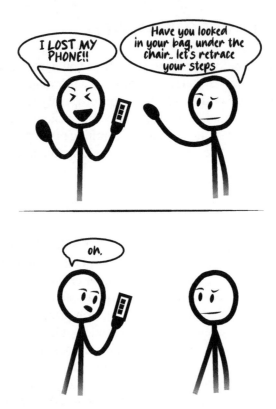

However, there are often external constraints, such as the scope of your project, available time and resources, which mean that a proportion of rather than all the evidence on a subject needs to be sourced. To ensure you understand what is required, complete the next checkpoint activity.

 Aim: To clarify the expectations of finding articles for your assignment and if a discussion of this process is a requirement of the assignment.

Instructions: As explained in Chapter 3, not all EBP assessments will require students to find their own evidence to appraise. For example, you may be given the article(s) by your module team so you may not have to write about searching for evidence. In contrast, if you are expected to source your own paper(s), you may be required to include details of the importance of systematic searching to EBP and the process you embarked on to find the evidenced used in your assignment.

4.4   PREPARE TO BE FRUSTRATED!

Searching may seem straightforward, but developing a search strategy is a commonly a frustrating exercise (Aveyard 2019). So before we move any further forward with the steps required for conducting good searches, it is worth saying that this is not an easy process. Lots of people find this a very difficult stage to action and students often struggle to describe it sufficiently in their assignments to convince their markers that they did it correctly. What is perhaps misleading is that in published literature reviews authors present their search methods in a concise and linear way, but for many (or most) the early stages of the search would not have been like this. People who conduct reviews can spend months getting the methods correct, actioning lots of different searches on different databases, making mistakes and trying again. The reason for this difficulty is that the leading question, or topic area, is not yet defined enough to develop a rigorous and repeatable search. At this early stage, the focus of the search keeps shifting, often without the person conducting the search really being aware of it.

A reason that students commonly become frustrated with searching is that they do not action the steps of the search in a sequenced way. For example, when searching it is common to get distracted by papers that are interesting but not relevant, or to follow the trail of linked papers and citation lists, or search terms may be added or changed and soon several hours have passed with little to show for it. Worse still, if you take a break from searching, you may return to find you have been logged out of the database and your search history has been deleted. We helpfully explain how to avoid these problems later in the chapter.

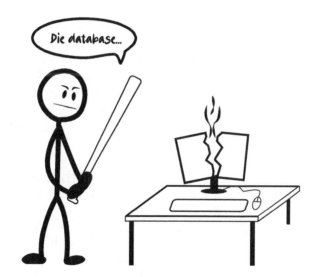

4.5   LOOKING FOR THE EVIDENCE

The reason for and topic of your search will determine where you look for your evidence. There are a range of evidence sources for you to use, and each has its own strengths and weaknesses. There are lots of different sources you will use for an assignment. Some are easier to read and access then others. Students, especially early on in their studies, tend to focus on books and websites. Such material is generally easy to access and understand. However, textbooks date quickly and it is not always possible to determine if the website you are using is sufficiently rigorous. For example, it is not always clear when the website was last updated, who it was written by, and if anyone beyond the developers checks the content is correct. Adding to the challenge of using websites is that there are usually so many results to review that it is impossible to know if you are using the best ones.

The quality of online materials varies enormously, so always think carefully before using them (De Brún and Pearce-Smith 2014). If we take information on personal websites, for example, much of it is speculative and subjective. It can also be very one-sided or, worse, misleading. Organisational websites are better, but often it is not clear how information is fact-checked or updated and, depending on the organisation, the information may be biased in its views. There are more credible websites such as those of the National Institute for Health and Care Excellence (NICE; www.nice.org.uk) and the Scottish Intercollegiate Guidelines Network (SIGN; www.sign.ac.uk). However, it is the evidence on these websites, rather than the website itself, that is of primary interest; that is, it is the report, review, or guideline that is most important to practice. Further to this there are organisations like the Cochrane Collaboration that conduct large reviews of research in healthcare and health policy to inform clinical decision-making. Cochrane Reviews are particularly important sources of pre-appraised evidence.

As you progress through your studies, you should be accessing professional journals. These journals are an excellent resource to inform practice, publishing a range of articles like reflections, expert opinions, and different types of research. Often these are written in a communicative and accessible language and will interpret some of the leading evidence specifically for health professionals who are unlikely, or unable, to access the study itself. In addition, these journals often publish small-scale pilots, feasibility studies, and student research and provide a really useful indication of topics that are important to today's practice.

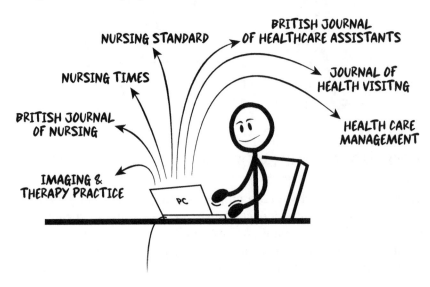

Despite the many advantages of professional journals, for more significant and larger-scale research you need to look in more academic or 'high-impact' journals. These are influential publications with good standing in their field of interest.

 Research Essentials

Impact factor: 'The impact factor, a simple mathematical formula reflecting the number of citations of a journal's material divided by the number of citable materials published by that same journal, has evolved to become one of the most influential tools in modern research and academia' (Kurmis 2003, p. 2449).

In contrast, professional journals often have low impact factors or none at all. In Table 4.1 you can see impact factors of some of the leading journals in nursing. Compare these to the *British Medical Journal*, which at the time of writing cites an impact factor of 30.223.

 Explore It

Why don't you investigate the impact factors of journals you commonly use in your discipline? These are usually reported on the journal home page. Or search for the journal online and add 'impact factor' to the online search bar. You should then be directed to its published impact factor for the current year.

TABLE 4.1   Impact factors of nursing journals.

Journal	Impact factor[a]
International Journal of Nursing Studies	8.1
Journal of Advanced Nursing	3.8
Nurse Education Today	3.9
Journal of Clinical Nursing	4.2
Nurse Education in Practice	3.2
Nursing Times	0
Nursing Standard	0
British Journal of Nursing	0

[a] At the time of publication; these usually fluctuate each year.

The disadvantage of using many of these higher-impact journals is that they are often written in a tone and style that many students find inaccessible. In addition, students can find the methods confusing and the findings difficult to interpret. However, it is these studies that can really influence practice (hence the 'high impact') and therefore you need to be able to find and use research published in these sorts of journals. Don't worry, though: Chapter 5 explains the structure of these kinds of articles so you can feel more confident about using them.

It is also worth pointing out that 'high impact' does not always mean 'high quality'. Poor research may be published in high-impact journals and good research published in low-impact journals. It is your job to evaluate the merits and limitations of a particular study. However, understanding the difference between journals is important, so do not over-rely on those you find easy to access and understand.

4.5.1   Peer-Reviewed Journal Articles

For an article to be published in a journal, it is usually reviewed either by an editorial board or via a peer review process.

 Research Essentials

Definition of peer review: 'Reviewers play a pivotal role in scholarly publishing. The peer review system exists to validate academic work, helps to improve the quality of published research, and increases networking possibilities within research communities. Despite criticisms, peer review is still the only widely accepted method for research validation and has continued successfully with relatively minor changes for some 350 years' (Elsevier 2023).

Peer reviewers are normally considered experts in the field and so are relied on to have a good knowledge base of the topic area under review. Peer review can be blind (reviewers and/or authors remain anonymous) or open (reviewers and authors are known to each other) and there are pros and cons to both approaches. Usually, the higher-impact journals have a more stringent peer review process, and lower-impact journals tend to be more flexible and less detailed. This is why higher-impact journals often allow a higher word count, because they require more detailed reporting. Through the peer review process authors will typically be asked to make revisions before their work is published. Some journals like *BMJ Open* even publish the reviews so you can see the history of the manuscript and the revisions made.

The peer review process means that readers can be more confident about the quality and accuracy of the information presented. However, peer reviewers can miss things, make mistakes, or be biased in their reviews. There are some very high-profile examples of poor research that was peer reviewed before publication in a high-impact journal. One of the most well-known examples is a paper that incorrectly identified a link between MMR immunisation and autism in children. It was published in *The Lancet*, a very prestigious medical journal, and many serious flaws related to both the research methods and ethical issues were missed. Although it was subsequently retracted, it was widely read and contributed to a decline in vaccination rates (Eggertson 2010). So peer review means it is more likely that the evidence presented is accurate and good quality, but it is not a guarantee. Health professionals must be able to appraise evidence themselves and apply a critical eye to every source they use.

 Explore It

Take a look at a paper by Eggertson (2010) on the retracted article that claimed a link between autism and MMR vaccines: `https://www.ncbi.nlm.nih.gov/pmc/articles/PMC2831678`
What views do you and people you know have on the MMR vaccine? How were these opinions formed? Have your views changed over the years or stayed the same?

4.5.2 Types of Journal Article

While journals will have preferences regarding the type of article they publish, you will generally find a range of discussion papers, editorials, and debates on contemporary issues alongside different types of primary and secondary research. Increasingly, researchers are also publishing study protocols, which are plans or proposals for a forthcoming study. These are published to support increased transparency of research and prevent duplication of studies, but to the uninitiated they can look very similar to a completed research study. It is not uncommon for a student to think they have a research paper when actually it is a discussion paper or a protocol. To add to this, there are journals like *Evidence Based Nursing* that publish commentaries on research. While these are excellent at helping to guide decision-making when applying evidence, they are not research evidence in themselves. So it remains important for students to become proficient at locating and appraising completed research studies.

Table 4.2 identifies common types of journal articles and describes their key features. There is more on understanding the type of research you are appraising in Chapters 5 and 6.

4.6 HOW TO FIND RESEARCH

4.6.1 Searching for Research

Finding research is relatively easy these days. Most journals have their own websites and research is increasingly 'open access', meaning anyone, anywhere can read the final published manuscript in full and free of charge. Other research is made open

TABLE 4.2   Common types of journal article.

Publication type	Subcategory	Content	Key features
Research	Primary	Qualitative Quantitative Mixed	Authors have recruited participants and collected their own data. They describe analysis and report results or findings.
	Secondary	Systematic review Integrative review Narrative review	Authors have followed a systematic process to retrieve research. Results are based on a synthesis of selected studies.
Abstracts	Any	Any	Short (200–300 words), structured or unstructured summaries of studies in progress or complete. Abstracts may be related to conference proceedings and are indicative of interest in specific topics and of future publications.
Protocols	Primary/ secondary	Planned methods for a future study.	Detailed account of methods but no participants recruited, nor results reported.
Opinion pieces	Editorials	Editor's opinion on an issue relevant to the journal.	Raising awareness of a particular issue, may be provocative or persuasive to prompt discussion and debate. Often unstructured.
	Discussion papers Contemporary issues for debate	Authors provide their perspective or experience of a topic relevant to the journal's readership.	Structured debate, but no participants, no data, no results.

access through publishing pre-print copies on platforms such as ResearchGate (www.researchgate.net) or university online research archives. Despite this, a large amount of research is only available if you pay for it. For students, many of these fees are paid by your university through a site-wide licence for specific journals. This normally means you need to use your institutional passwords to access these. Despite these licences, there will still be research that you cannot easily get hold of because different institutions pay for different licences depending on the needs of their student population. If you find an article you want but it appears that it can only be accessed by paying a fee, you can instead usually request it using a process called an 'inter-library loan'. This is a service whereby libraries work together to source and supply items for borrowers. This applies to journal publications as well as more traditional inter-library loans like books. These loans are often for a very small charge or free for certain groups of students. So speak to a librarian before you consider paying any journal the listed price for access to an article that you need.

In the context of EBP, it is important to source *all* the evidence on a topic, not just that which is easily accessible through the internet or your institution. Therefore, if you are conducting a literature review, you need to retrieve all the evidence on the topic in order to see the whole picture. If you do not take this approach and instead are selective about the evidence you source, it will lead to a biased and restricted view of the evidence base. Any findings or recommendations will thereby also be biased, and this is not a good outcome if you are engaging in the EBP process to lead decisions in professional practice.

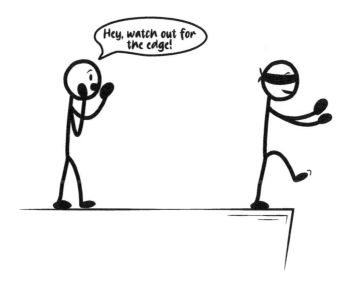

4.6.2 Internet Searching

In designing a search strategy, you need to decide where to search, how comprehensive you want to be, how much time you have, and how feasible the task is (Caldwell and Bennett 2020). We all love the internet and search engines like Google tend to be the first place people go when they need to know anything. Some trending questions on Google include: Why were cornflakes invented? Why is the sky blue? Why do dogs eat grass? Such questions prove our inquisitive nature, our desire for answers, and probably how easily distracted we are!

In the context of finding research, you are guaranteed results if you copy and paste your leading question into a search engine and press search. Results like this may quench your thirst for immediate results, but the results are usually too numerous and broad for you to review past the first few pages of results. Therefore, searching on an engine like Google is a bit like opening the window and shouting into the street.

Someone is bound to reply, but are they the right person, is this the information you need, is it filtered or quality checked?

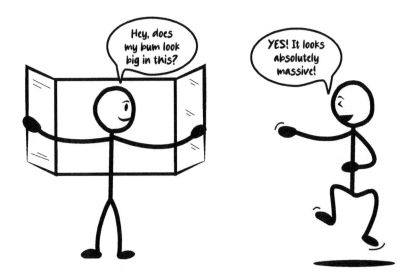

The other, and perhaps more concerning, issue with internet searching is 'search engine optimisation'. Despite you feeling in control of your search process, in fact algorithms are in control of the search result. That means that your results are based on your search history, your cookies, and your browser settings. So different people will have different results despite undertaking the same search. As mentioned earlier, for EBP you need a systematic and repeatable process, so that someone else can do the same search and get the same results and evidence to reach the same decisions. For a systematic and repeatable search, you need to be searching on *subject-specific databases*.

4.6.3   Subject-Specific Databases

A subject-specific database is a catalogue, or index, which contains hundreds of thousands of searchable items on a huge variety of topics.

 Explore It

Do you know what a healthcare database is? Can you name any healthcare databases? Do you know how to access healthcare databases? Have you ever used a healthcare database to retrieve a journal article?

If you have answered 'no' to any of these questions, spend some time on your university's library home page, where you will find helpful guides on what databases are most appropriate for your programme and how to use them. It would be worth doing this before progressing in this chapter.

Each subject area will have databases that house items of interest to that subject. For example, CINAHL (Cumulative Index of Nursing and Allied Health Literature) contains publications that are most relevant to nursing and allied health, whereas Medline and PubMed contain those publications that are most relevant to medicine. Given that both databases are about health there will of course be some overlap in the publications they index. However, there are always some publications that are specific only to the database being searched. This is why searching multiple databases is recommended. These databases are normally accessed through your university's library website and a subject librarian will be able to help you to use them. See Box 4.1 for other databases you may investigate.

It is worth mentioning that there are also *database host* services. Examples include EBSCO, OVID, and ProQuest. These platforms provide access to databases but are not databases themselves. Different institutions will use different host services to provide you with a gateway to the databases they subscribe to, so while the access route will differ, the database will remain the same. However, despite this, recent research has shown that the host service does make a difference to the search results. The benefit of using a host service is that even when you are searching in different databases, the search page will look and feel the same for the user. Furthermore, it is easier to copy a search from one database to another within the same host.

Box 4.1 Databases to Support Clinical and Non-clinical Decision-making

CINAHL (subscription only): Covers a wide range of topics including nursing, biomedicine, health sciences librarianship, alternative/complementary medicine, consumer health, and 17 allied health disciplines.

Cochrane Library (free) – `http://www.thecochranelibrary.com/view/0/index.html`: Six databases that contain different types of high-quality, independent evidence to inform healthcare decision-making.

Embase (subscription only): European version of Medline, containing abstracts of articles on medical and pharmacological research.

Medline (subscription only)/PubMed (free) – `www.pubmed.gov`: Medline and PubMed have the same content, made up of more than 22 million citations from biomedical literature.

NICE Evidence Search (free) – `http://www.evidence.nhs.uk`: Evidence Search provides free open access to a unique index of selected and authoritative health and social care evidence-based information.

Social Care Online (free) – `http://www.scie-socialcareonline.org.uk`: Largest database of information and research on all aspects of social care and social work.

TRIP Database (free) – `http://www.tripdatabase.com`: Clinical search engine designed to allow users to quickly and easily find and use high-quality research evidence to support their practice and/or care.

Information sourced from de Brún (2013).

Assignment Tip

When it comes to reporting your search process, report the individual databases that you searched and then state the host service you used to access them, e.g. 'Medline, CINAHL and Amed were searched through EBSCO host'.

In addition to the individual subject-specific databases, libraries often have their own database that combines subject-specific databases and enables you to complete combined searches. These are extremely useful when writing assignments, but when conducting a systematic search they are best avoided because they do not always allow you to develop or use an advanced search technique.

Assignment Tip

When conducting systematic searches for a literature review it is advisable to search each database separately. Although this may seem laborious, when creating a technical and complex search using features like truncation, syntax, parentheses, and database thesauruses (see later in this chapter), this can only be done within single databases.

4.6.4   Developing a Search Strategy

Instead of jumping straight into the search and expecting it to work first time, you need to spend some time thinking about and planning the search. Time spent thinking about how to search properly is time well spent (Aveyard 2019). Expect several iterations of this before you get it right. Having just been cautioned against Google searching, you may want to start with a quick scoping exercise using a search engine just to get an idea of what's out there. This starts to shape your thinking and helps you identify what the topic is and what you are not interested in.

In the next checkpoint activity we ask you to spend a little time on the internet testing out searches about your topic of interest. This process helps you develop a searchable question and its associated search terms, which can then be added to an EBP question framework as we will show later.

Checkpoint Activity   **Aim:** To complete a scoping exercise for a topic of interest.

Instructions: Conduct an internet search on your topic of interest. Use this time to reflect on areas that you are interested in and what you are not interested in. Make a note of any areas that you are yet to make your mind up about. You should write down any search terms that work well and those that do not. You can mind map this process like we have done in the next image or create your own.

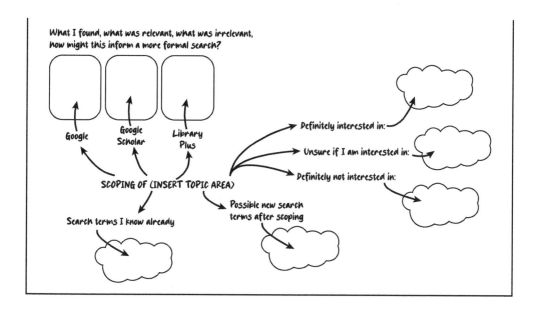

4.6.5 Systematic Searching

Moving from an informal, and quite relaxed, process of searching towards developing a systematic search strategy is not an easy step. Unless you conduct academic searches regularly, your skills of searching are most likely underdeveloped. Like all new skills, practice makes perfect! Often this is when help from an expert is required. Librarians are amazing sources of knowledge and expertise around systematic searching and they have skills in complex database searching and literature retrieval (McGowan 2012). Libraries often have a subject specialist and run sessions to help you develop and hone your systematic searching skills, so why not make an appointment?

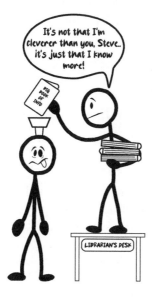

Now we explore some common problems students tell us they have when they attempt systematic searching.

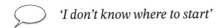 *'I don't know where to start'*

The first step in a systematic search strategy is to have a good question, one that is clear, defined, and focused. As was explained in Chapter 3, EBP starts with a relevant and well-designed question. As described earlier questions are often developed around frameworks such as PICO, PICOT, PIO, PEO, SPICE, and SPIDER. In order to conduct a systematic search, you first need to break your well-designed question down into its searchable components. This can be done according to the framework chosen by using the acronym to separate the concepts of interest and beginning to generate as many related search terms as possible (Wakefield 2015).

If you don't have a question designed in this way, you may still be able to isolate the different concepts of interest. However, be warned that unstructured questions are far less precise and will result in a much wider and less focused search. The result is often too many studies that are not related to what you are interested in. Therefore, you should always attempt a structured format, but apply some flexibility if the framework becomes restrictive.

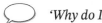 *'Why do I need lots of search terms?'*

Only very rarely should a review question be searched by relying on single search terms. Remember that in EBP you need to understand the full picture and not just part of it. So it is important to take into account that people may not all use the same language, spellings, or definitions to describe the phenomenon you are interested in. For example, you may be interested in children, but publications may refer to paediatric or pediatric, so you need the search to be as inclusive as possible to capture all these perspectives. This is called **high recall**.

 Research Essentials

High recall means that a search has been designed to capture all publications relevant to the topic.

Therefore, you need to search for synonyms that may be applied as well as the term you have used in your question. A simple example would be searching for 'healthcare assistant', 'health-care assistant' and also 'HCA'. These terms mean the same and authors may have used any in their paper, so you must build a search that prepares for all eventualities. For a search to be considered comprehensive, all the different terms, spellings, and acronyms must be built into the search strategy (De Brún and Pearce-Smith 2014).

In addition to this you may also need to incorporate truncation, wild cards, and quotation marks. These are useful shortcuts that help to reduce the number of search terms you need to add to the database. Truncation is used to shorten a search term by adding an asterisk * or dollar sign $ to a word or part of one, which will enable the database to search for alternative endings. An example of this would be Nurs*, which would search for nurse, nurses, and nursing. However, always be careful, as such a search would also include nursery, which may or may not be relevant to your search.

Wildcards can be used in the middle of words and are useful for different spellings or plurals. Often the symbol is a question mark, so if you were interested in women or woman you could use wom?n, or an?mia would facilitate a search with both American and British English spellings of this condition (you will need to check what each database uses). Finally, the use of speech marks is helpful in searches as it tells the database to search for an *exact phrase* ("healthcare professional") and not the terms independently of each other.

You should now be able to create search terms using an EBP question framework, as shown in the next activity.

 Aim: To use an EBP question framework to develop database search terms.

Instructions: Draw a table like the one that follows. Add your EBP question framework to the column headings. In the next row identify each of the main concepts and underneath write down any synonyms that relate to these. If you need some help, look at our example based on PEO (population, exposure, outcome).

EBP question framework				
Concept				
Synonyms				

EBP question framework	Population	Exposure	Outcome
Concept	Nursing	Lifting	Pain
Synonyms	Nurs*	Manual handling Moving Patient load "Moving and handling"	Injury "Back pain" Trauma "Chronic pain"

 'What is free-text searching?'

The best database searches are carefully constructed layer by layer, which means searches being conducted simply and precisely. To do this, it is better to search for each key term individually and then combine them in a later stage of the search process.

FIGURE 4.1 How to select a field to restrict a search.

Adding search terms to a database as described in the checkpoint activity is known as a 'free-text' search. Such searches are not restricted in any way, so as long as your search term is somewhere in the paper it will appear in your results list. For some searches this is not a problem, but when the term is broad like 'care' a free-text search will result in thousands of results, many of which will be irrelevant to the act of care in a professional context. To increase relevance and reduce the number of results you can limit the search by specific fields. Limits can be chosen from the drop-down menu next to the search box (see Figure 4.1).

The most useful limit here is to limit by abstract, so your search term must be mentioned in the abstract to be retrieved in your results. Of course, an unwelcome consequence of reducing your results is that you may miss key papers. Therefore, an effective counterweight to using such limits is to use a database thesaurus (De Brún and Pearce-Smith 2014).

'What is a database thesaurus?'

A database thesaurus search is an advanced search technique that uses the subject terms (also called controlled vocabulary) that the particular database assigns to a paper so that it can index it properly. Think of this like a filing cabinet. When a paper is published it is filed according to the system being used by that database. Each database may therefore have a different thesaurus. In Medline this is called a MESH term or 'Medical Subject Heading', in CINAHL a 'CINAHL Subject Heading'. When you select a search term from the thesaurus it will automatically include different spellings, plurals, acronyms, and related terms.

Looking in the thesauruses of databases in the exploratory phase of designing your search strategy can actually help to identify synonyms, which spelling to use, and what combinations of terms are most commonly used. However, thesaurus searching can become quite complex, so if you want to use this more advanced technique you would do well to take advice from a librarian.

'Can I just use one database?'

It is recommended that searches are conducted on multiple databases to reduce the likelihood of missing relevant papers (Caldwell and Bennett 2020). Although most people will have a favourite database, you should start with the database you are confident will retrieve most of the relevant literature on the topic of interest. Once you have a plan for your search and are confident that you have identified the key concepts relevant to your question, you are ready to start conducting a search in that database. With the exception of thesaurus searching, the process of database searching is much the same between databases. Therefore, once you have mastered searching in one database you can transfer these skills to another one.

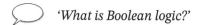 'How can I avoid having too many results?'

High-recall searches will capture a lot of results, many of which are completely irrelevant. Therefore, the searching process must progress to what is called **high precision**.

 Research Essentials

High precision means that the search, and its results, are very closely related to the question you want to answer because they include all of the key concepts relevant to your question.

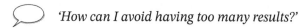 'What is Boolean logic?'

In databases you will see the option to combine searches using AND, OR, and NOT. This is called 'Boolean logic' and enables you to develop your own high-recall and high-precision searches. This combining of searches using Boolean logic is illustrated in Figure 4.2.

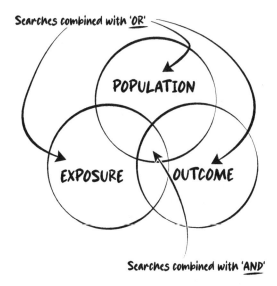

FIGURE 4.2 How Boolean logic works.

As mentioned previously, it is good practice to conduct searches using individual search terms one at a time. If you just add lots of search terms to the search box, like 'Occupational therapy OR Nurse OR Radiographer', it is not always easy to see that you may have spelt a key word incorrectly or made some other error like not using quotes around the words "occupational therapy". Such errors will lead to frustration and poor results later on. If searches are conducted individually, they can be deleted or edited and rerun, so the search is easily improved and revised as you become more confident. Again, this will feel like a laborious first step, but as you build up your skills each stage will become quicker, more intuitive, and lead to more successful searches overall.

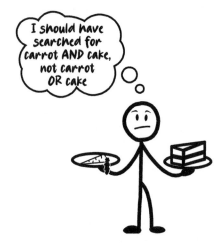

The first Boolean operator we use is 'OR'. Using OR allows us to combine searches of similar and related terms. If you refer back to the search terms and synonyms in the Checkpoint Activity, you can see columns of related terms. These searches need to be combined for high recall of papers related to the concept of interest. You will then generate a search that combines all related key words with OR. As a high-recall search, you can expect retrieval to be wide and broad. See Figure 4.3 for how OR is used in a high-recall search.

Next, we need to move from high recall to high precision, whereby the results retrieved contain all of the key terms related to the question, just like in Figure 4.2. This is where we need to use the Boolean operator 'AND'. This is illustrated in the final line of Figure 4.4.

Lastly, we can use the Boolean operator 'NOT'. NOT can be added to identify publications that you definitely do not want to retrieve in your search, for example 'diabetes NOT insipidus'. However, use it sparingly and with caution, if at all, as you run the risk of excluding papers that are relevant to your question. Therefore, more commonly NOT is not used in search strategies.

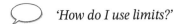 *'How do I use limits?'*

The next stage is to apply limits to the final search. Databases differ in the limits that are available but most have limits like year of publication, peer reviewed, English

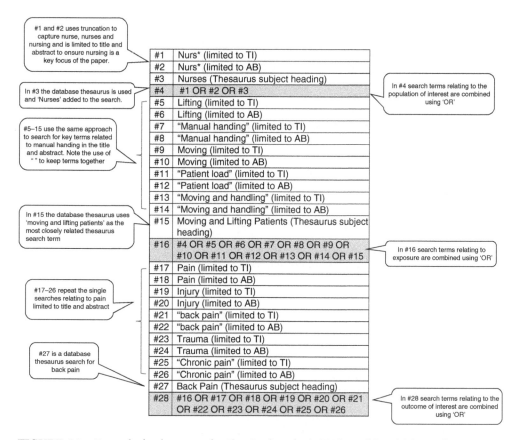

#1	Nurs* (limited to TI)
#2	Nurs* (limited to AB)
#3	Nurses (Thesaurus subject heading)
#4	#1 OR #2 OR #3
#5	Lifting (limited to TI)
#6	Lifting (limited to AB)
#7	"Manual handing" (limited to TI)
#8	"Manual handing" (limited to AB)
#9	Moving (limited to TI)
#10	Moving (limited to AB)
#11	"Patient load" (limited to TI)
#12	"Patient load" (limited to AB)
#13	"Moving and handling" (limited to TI)
#14	"Moving and handling" (limited to AB)
#15	Moving and Lifting Patients (Thesaurus subject heading)
#16	#4 OR #5 OR #6 OR #7 OR #8 OR #9 OR #10 OR #11 OR #12 OR #13 OR #14 OR #15
#17	Pain (limited to TI)
#18	Pain (limited to AB)
#19	Injury (limited to TI)
#20	Injury (limited to AB)
#21	"back pain" (limited to TI)
#22	"back pain" (limited to AB)
#23	Trauma (limited to TI)
#24	Trauma (limited to AB)
#25	"Chronic pain" (limited to TI)
#26	"Chronic pain" (limited to AB)
#27	Back Pain (Thesaurus subject heading)
#28	#16 OR #17 OR #18 OR #19 OR #20 OR #21 OR #22 OR #23 OR #24 OR #25 OR #26

#1 and #2 uses truncation to capture nurse, nurses and nursing and is limited to title and abstract to ensure nursing is a key focus of the paper.

In #3 the database thesaurus is used and 'Nurses' added to the search.

In #4 search terms relating to the population of interest are combined using 'OR'

#5–15 use the same approach to search for key terms related to manual handing in the title and abstract. Note the use of " " to keep terms together

In #15 the database thesaurus uses 'moving and lifting patients' as the most closely related thesaurus search term

In #16 search terms relating to exposure are combined using 'OR'

#17–26 repeat the single searches relating to pain limited to title and abstract

#27 is a database thesaurus search for back pain

In #28 search terms relating to the outcome of interest are combined using 'OR'

FIGURE 4.3 Example database search using Boolean logic 'OR' to achieve high recall.

language. Once again, use these sparingly and with a good deal of thought about the implications for your search. One limit that students like at this stage is to 'limit by full text'. Limiting in this way means all the citations retrieved come with links to the full text. This is a pragmatic search feature that reduces time and effort when writing an assignment. However, if you are completing a systematic search, **do not limit by full text**. It will bias your search in relation to those that are available at your institution, and so will not be comprehensive or objective. It is unlikely this limit would ever be acceptable in the context of a systematic search, so you will need to access these publications through your library's inter-library loan service, as discussed earlier. This rule may differ within the context of your assignment, so talk with your module leader about the expectations for your module.

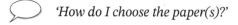

'How do I choose the paper(s)?'

Now you are ready to review your results and decide which citations are relevant and which are not. This can be done relatively quickly through a review of titles and abstracts. At this stage resist the urge to open the full text and look at the paper in detail. Instead, if you are using EBSCO host you can add citations of interest to a folder to look at once

#1	Nurs* (limited to TI)
#2	Nurs* (limited to AB)
#3	Nurses (Thesaurus subject heading)
#4	#1 OR #2 OR #3
#5	Lifting (limited to TI)
#6	Lifting (limited to AB)
#7	"Manual handing" (limited to TI)
#8	"Manual handing" (limited to AB)
#9	Moving (limited to TI)
#10	Moving (limited to AB)
#11	"Patient load" (limited to TI)
#12	"Patient load" (limited to AB)
#13	"Moving and handling" (limited to TI)
#14	"Moving and handling" (limited to AB)
#15	Moving and Lifting Patients (Thesaurus subject heading)
#16	#4 OR #5 OR #6 OR #7 OR #8 OR #9 OR #10 OR #11 OR #12 OR #13 OR #14 OR #15
#17	Pain (limited to TI)
#18	Pain (limited to AB)
#19	Injury (limited to TI)
#20	Injury (limited to AB)
#21	"back pain" (limited to TI)
#22	"back pain" (limited to AB)
#23	Trauma (limited to TI)
#24	Trauma (limited to AB)
#25	"Chronic pain" (limited to TI)
#26	"Chronic pain" (limited to AB)
#27	Back Pain (Thesaurus subject heading)
#28	#16 OR #17 OR #18 OR #19 OR #20 OR #21 OR #22 OR #23 OR #24 OR #25 OR #26
#29	#4 AND #15 AND #27

In #29 the 'OR' searches are combined with 'AND'

FIGURE 4.4   Example database search using Boolean logic 'AND' to achieve high precision.

you have reviewed the titles and abstracts of all the papers in your results list. To use folders in the databases you need to register for an account, which is free and easy to do. Another benefit of registering for an account is that you can save searches and receive alerts if new papers are published that match your search criteria. Using folders and saved searches means your searches are available for when you need to write up your review methods (Bettany-Saltikov 2012). If using other host services such as Ovid the folder function may not be available, so you may want to use reference management software or simply take notes and copy titles into a Microsoft Word document.

Once you have reviewed all the results and have a folder or document with papers that look like they should be relevant to your review question, you can start to 'review by full text'. Again, be really focused on completing this stage to filter papers that do and do not address your review question. If there are interesting papers that are not relevant, make a note of the citation details before removing them so you can retrieve them again later on.

TABLE 4.3 Example of inclusion and exclusion criteria used in a systematic search.

Inclusion	Exclusion
English language	Pre-2010
Peer reviewed	Doctoral theses
Primary research	Conference abstracts

It is important to remember that this selection of papers is an active process, in which you are in control of the decision-making. If someone else was trying to repeat the same search they would need the criteria you used to include or exclude papers. So you need to make a note of the reasons why you kept papers and why you decided to remove citations you first thought were relevant (Wakefield 2015). You should then be able to list these as inclusion and exclusion criteria. A table of these is usually required when writing up methods of searching. An example is included in Table 4.3 with some generic inclusion and exclusion criteria that may be relevant to your search strategy. However, you should also develop some that are specific to your question, like include adult, exclude children and adolescents.

 Assignment Tip

If you are expected to write about your search strategy in your assignment you may want to include:

- A rationale for the chosen databases.
- An account of how the EBP question framework was used to develop search terms and how these were actioned.
- How Boolean operators facilitate both high-recall and high-precision searches.
- A justification for the selected paper(s).

 'Can I look elsewhere?'

It is important to remember that despite your best efforts in the databases, you may still miss important literature. In addition, not all literature may be indexed in the databases you searched. So a comprehensive search strategy will include complementary searches too.

 'What are complementary searches?'

As the name suggests, complementary searches balance systematic and focused searches on databases to check that nothing has been missed. It is important to remember that complementary searching is a 'mop-up' of any final papers that are relevant to your review. If you retrieve more papers in these searches than you did in the database searching, this implies a poor search strategy, so you may need to revise your search strategy and redo the search with some additional search terms.

Citation searches, hand searches, and internet searches complete the search process. Citation searches are where you look at the reference list of papers you have chosen to include in your review. Sometimes students think this is 'cheating', but it is all part of making sure you haven't missed anything. To add to this, more people are conducting 'citation forward' searches, which is looking at papers that have cited the papers retrieved from the databases and is another useful tactic to trace important papers. The inclusion of 'hand searching' is where you look at the contents lists of key journals that are relevant to your topic of interest. Finally, you may wish to include a Google Scholar search to source any final papers that did not come up in the databases.

In some types of reviews, it is important, or expected, to source what is known as 'grey literature'. Grey literature is evidence that is often in the public domain, but is not published in commercial journals. There are many different types of grey literature that may be relevant to a systematic review, including theses, dissertations, reports, conference papers, and abstracts. These are rich sources of evidence that can counteract some of the publication bias seen in journals that may have a preference for particular types of studies and those that report only positive findings (Paez 2017).

While bigger systematic reviews will often source grey literature, the expectation that students will use this for their extended piece of work can vary, so it is important to check the assessment requirements with your module team. If you are required to look for grey literature it cannot all be found in the databases because grey literature is not published in journals. Therefore, you need a different way to look for this, usually by accessing specific websites. A similar search to the one actioned in the databases can then be conducted here, but it may have to be a simplified version as these websites do not always have advanced search features. A list of useful sources of grey literature is given in Box 4.2.

Box 4.2   Sources of Grey Literature

- http://www.opengrey.eu
- https://wonder.cdc.gov
- http://www.opengrey.eu
- https://search.proquest.com/cpi
- https://clinicaltrials.gov
- https://www.evidence.nhs.uk
- https://www.scie-socialcareonline.org.uk
- https://www.who.int/clinical-trials-registry-platform

4.7 TRANSPARENT REPORTING OF SEARCH METHODS

Search methods should be reported clearly enough to enable the reader to judge if the methods were robust and steps actioned appropriately. While you may not be trying to publish your search in an academic journal, the Preferred Reporting Items for Systematic Reviews and Meta-Analyses (PRISMA) checklist demonstrates what authors typically include in their manuscript if they want to publish their literature review.

 Explore It

Take a look at the PRISMA checklist. How might this help you in your assignments?

```
http://prisma-statement.org/prismastatement/Checklist.aspx
```

 Assignment Tip

If you are expected to write about your search strategy in your assignment, you may want to include some of the items on the PRISMA checklist, such as:

- Specify inclusion and exclusion criteria with rationale.
- Describe all databases used and other ways information was sourced like citation searches, hand searches, internet searches. Include first and last date searched.
- Present full electronic search strategy for at least one database, including any limits used, such that it could be repeated.
- Give numbers of studies screened, assessed for eligibility and included in the review, with reasons for exclusions at each stage.

In addition to the checklist, PRISMA provides a useful flowchart of key milestones in the selection of papers in a literature review. Milestones include the number of results achieved in the database searches, the number of papers removed following review by title and abstract, the number removed following full-text review (with reasons for exclusion cited), and then finally the number of papers included in the review (Figure 4.5).

Therefore, in each of the stages of the search process, make a note of how many papers you identify for possible inclusion in the review.

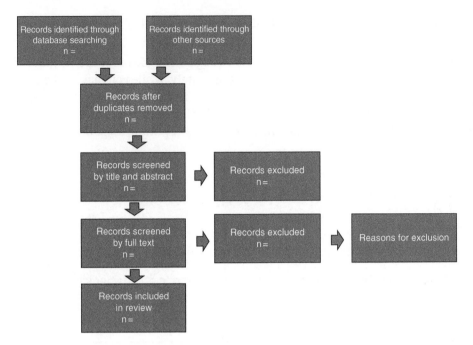

FIGURE 4.5 Flow chart for evidence acquisition based on the PRISMA guidelines.

4.8 WRITING ABOUT SYSTEMATIC SEARCHING IN YOUR ASSIGNMENT

Your assignment may not require you to search for your own evidence; however, it may still be important to demonstrate that you understand the principles and importance of systematic searching. Systematically searching for evidence is a key part of the EBP process, so consider including a brief discussion of appropriate database choices, question frameworks, or reducing bias when filtering and selecting studies.

If writing about the search process is an expected part of your assignment, take care not to simply describe it. Use of tables and figures will help with the detailed account of the methods employed, and these can be presented in appendices or in the main text depending on your assignment brief.

Make writing more analytical by discussing the key stages of the search process, why these are important, and any reflections on how they were actioned in your search. Use a few different sources so that you can include different perspectives.

4.9 ASSIGNMENT EXAMPLES

Example 1: De Brún (2013) says finding evidence begins by asking an answerable question, then identifying synonyms and developing a search strategy and identifying appropriate information sources, followed by searching for evidence and appraising the results. Databases like PubMed, Google Scholar and the Cochrane Library can be used to search for evidence, using keywords. Aromataris and Riitano (2014) say search strategies are important to ensure you find a good range of evidence specific to the search and not too limited that crucial data is missed. Selçuk (2019) says PRISMA standardises systematic reviews and reduces bias. Moreover, the recent revision to PRISMA 2020 enables more transparency and accuracy with systematic reviews (Page et al. 2021).

Example 2: The electronic databases used in this literature review are Cumulative Index to Nursing and Allied Health Literature (CINAHL), Excerpta Medica Database (EMBASE) and Medical Literature Analysis and Retrieval System Online (MED-LINE). Aveyard (2019) recommends that CINAHL is an appropriate start when undertaking a literature review as it covers a vast range of international nursing literature. However, solely relying on the search results of one database may not provide sufficient evidence to answer the research question (Ellis 2019).

Utilising Boolean operators in the advanced search selection narrowed the literature down. Boolean operators include 'AND', 'OR' and 'NOT' commands to obtain refined literature applicable to the research question (Aromataris and Riitano 2014). According to Aveyard (2019), the 'AND' command links key terms to narrow down a search, finding literature containing several key terms, 'OR' command broadens a search and allows for several different terms or synonyms and 'NOT' excludes key terms; however, this should be used with caution as it can potentially exclude valid literature.

Identifying inclusion and exclusion criteria enabled the retrieval of relevant literature from the search results and to filter out irrelevant literature (Aveyard 2019). Parahoo (2014) explains that inclusion and exclusion criteria may affect the findings if the criteria are not justified. For example, having the inclusion criteria of peer-reviewed articles meant that studies retrieved were credible and valid. Additionally, collecting research focused primarily on males or including a male's voice separately were paramount to answering this literature review question.

4.10   END-OF-CHAPTER CHECKPOINT

		Comment/notes
I can access a healthcare database	Yes/no	
My preferred database is	....	
I have completed a table of search terms with synonyms, truncation, and wild cards	Yes/no	
I have conducted a simple database search using Boolean operators OR/AND	Yes/no	
I have conducted an advanced database search using truncation, limits, and the database thesaurus	Yes/no	

		Comment/notes
I know what grey literature is, how to search for it, and if I need to include it in my assignment	Yes/no	
I know who to contact at my university for support with my search strategy	Yes/no	
I have looked at the PRISMA guidelines	Yes/no	
I can list inclusion and exclusion criteria	Yes/no	
I know how to use folders and save searches in the databases	Yes/no	
I know how to write about my search strategy	Yes/no	

On a scale of 1–5, how confident do you feel about the content in this chapter?

4.11 CHAPTER SUMMARY

In this chapter we have introduced the importance of the systematic identification and retrieval of literature to underpin EBP. We have described the key features of systematic searching and how to use healthcare databases. We have explained that while systematic searching can be frustrating, searching skills must be mastered if you are to be an evidence-based practitioner. We would now recommend that you spend some time practising the techniques outlined in this chapter so that you can develop more confidence that you are retrieving relevant, contemporary research.

REFERENCES

Aromataris, E. and Riitano, D. (2014). Constructing a search strategy and searching for evidence. A guide to the literature search for a systematic review. *American Journal of Nursing* 114 (5): 49–56. https://doi.org/10.1097/01.NAJ.0000446779.99522.f6.

Aveyard, H. (2019). *Doing a Literature Review in Health and Social Care: A Practical Guide*, 4e. London: Open University Press.

Bettany-Saltikov, J. (2012). *How to Do a Systematic Literature Review in Nursing: A Step-by-Step Guide*, 2e. Maidenhead: Open University Press.

Caldwell, P.H. and Bennett, T. (2020). Easy guide to conducting a systematic review. *Journal of Paediatrics and Child Health* 56 (6): 853–856. https://doi.org/10.1111/jpc.14853.

Davis, D. (2016). A practical overview of how to conduct a systematic review. *Nursing Standard* 31: 60–71.

De Brún, C. (2013). Useful databases. *The Information Standard*, September. https://www.england.nhs.uk/tis/wp-content/uploads/sites/17/2014/09/tis-evidence-wrkshp-caroline-de-brun.pdf (accessed 4 December 2023).

De Brún, C. and Pearce-Smith, N. (2014). *Searching Skills Toolkit: Finding the Evidence*, 2e. Chichester: Wiley Blackwell.

Eggertson, L. (2010). Lancet retracts 12-year-old article linking autism to MMR vaccines. *Canadian Medical Association Journal* 182 (4): E199–E200. https://doi.org/10.1503/cmaj.109-3179.

Ellis, P. (2019). *Evidence Based Practice in Nursing*. London: Sage.

Elsevier (2023). What is peer review? https://www.elsevier.com/reviewers/what-is-peer-review.

Harari, M.B., Parola, H.R., Hartwell, C.J., and Riegelman, A. (2020). Literature searches in systematic reviews and meta-analyses: a review, evaluation, and recommendations. *Journal of Vocational Behavior* 118: 103377. https://doi.org/10.1016/j.jvb.2020.103377.

Kurmis, A.P. (2003). Understanding the limitations of the journal impact factor. *Journal of Bone and Joint Surgery* 85 (12): 2449–2454. https://doi.org/10.2106/00004623-200312000-00028.

McGowan, L. (2012). Systematic reviews: the good, the not so good and the good again. *British Journal of Midwifery* 20 (8): 588–592.

Paez, A. (2017). Grey literature: an important resource in systematic reviews. *Journal of Evidence-Based Medicine* https://doi.org/10.1111/jebm.12265.

Page, M.J., McKenzie, J.E., Bossuyt, P.M. et al. (2021). The PRISMA 2020 statement: an updated guideline for reporting systematic reviews. *BMJ (Clinical Research Ed.)* 372: n71. https://doi.org/10.1136/bmj.n71.

Parahoo, K. (2014). *Nursing Research: Principles, Process and Issues*. London: Bloomsbury.

Selçuk, A.A. (2019). A guide for systematic reviews: PRISMA. *Turkish Archives of Otorhinolaryngology* 57 (1): 57–58. https://doi.org/10.5152/tao.2019.4058.

Wakefield, A. (2015). Synthesising the literature as part of a literature review. *Nursing Standard* 29: 44–51.

CHAPTER 5

Preparing the Ground for Appraisal

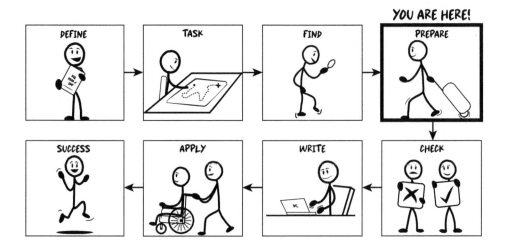

FIVE THINGS TO LEARN FROM THIS CHAPTER

1. It is common to feel confused, overwhelmed, and anxious about appraising a research study for an assignment – but there are ways to make it easier!
2. Appraisal is easier if you are familiar with the structure of research papers.

Critical Appraisal Skills for Healthcare Students: A Practical Guide to Writing Evidence-based Practice Assignments, First Edition. Charlotte J. Whiffin, Donna Barnes, and Lorraine Henshaw.
© 2024 John Wiley & Sons Ltd. Published 2024 by John Wiley & Sons Ltd.

3. Appraisal is easier if you understand the research process.
4. Appraisal is easier when you know what should be reported.
5. Appraisal is easier when you break it down into smaller steps.

FIVE MINUTES WITH JADE, MENTAL HEALTH NURSING STUDENT

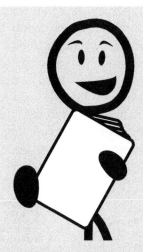

What do you think helped you succeed in your EBP module?
I strongly believe that selecting the right article was key to me doing well during this module. I had chosen a different study during the earlier weeks, but as I progressed through the weeks, I realised that the article was not suitable for me to critically analyse.

Having a system was essential for me, for example, working out when I was going to study, starting early, and bringing forward my deadline in case of any last-minute panics with the kids

What would you recommend other students do at the start of an EBP module?
Understand your learning outcomes and follow your assignment guidance. Definitely look at examples of critical appraisal as it will give you a better insight into what is expected. Choose a study early on, read the materials given and attend lessons!

Do you have any other advice to help other students do well?
Ask questions when in doubt.

Speak to your university library, as the university I attended held online courses to help with all different types of academic writing and different sections of assignments/dissertations.

5.1   INTRODUCTION

It's very common for students to feel anxious about starting research modules. It is not a new issue, nor is it restricted to healthcare students. Studies suggest that research assignment anxiety is experienced by students in many different countries and working in different fields (Papanastasiou and Zembylas 2008; Earley 2014). There are various contributing factors, but often the anxiety relates to misconceptions about research (Ramsay et al. 2020), perceptions that the teaching material will be too difficult, and concerns that the topic does not apply to students' professional roles (Earley 2014). Our own teaching experience suggests that anxiety also comes from students' lack of familiarity with reading research articles. Prior to a research or EBP module, students may have only read parts of a research study, for example the abstract or main findings. So research modules can feel more challenging because students are trying to learn about several different things at the same time – what research is, the various research designs and methods, what appraisal is, *and* the content of the actual research paper. No wonder it feels overwhelming and confusing!

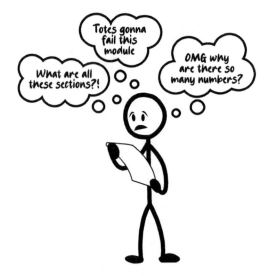

But help is at hand! This chapter provides practical strategies and tips to gradually build familiarity with how research articles are presented, what the different sections of a research article mean, and how appraisal can be broken down into more manageable steps. This advice will encourage a gradual and visible progression that will help to reduce anxiety and may even make it an enjoyable assignment process!

5.2   FINDING YOUR WAY AROUND A RESEARCH PAPER

To develop familiarity with published research, the first step is to look at as much of it as you can. You can do this when you are searching for a study to appraise for your assignment. Or if you are given a study to appraise by your tutor, you can do this when you are searching for other evidence on your study topic. As you look at more studies, you will see a wide variety in the layout, amount of detail, and formatting across different journals. Each journal has its own style and format guidelines. As shown in Figure 5.1, some studies are presented with clear headings and subheadings, and key details boxed separately, bullet pointed, or emphasised in some way. Others have several different elements of the study (the design and methods for example) presented as one block of writing. This does not mean the quality is different in either study, but for the task of appraising, an unclear layout can make it tricky to identify which part of the study is being described, particularly for those new to research. If you can choose your own study to appraise, pay attention to layout and how easily you are able to identify the different study elements from it.

As you look at more published research, you may then go on to notice that there is a standard order in which the key aspects of the study are reported. This order is

---

294   Journal of Blatantly Brilliant Research

Research Article

Study of healthcare student enjoyment of research assignments

D. Barnes

Abstract
Lorem ipsum dolor sit amet, consectetur adipiscing elit. Nam tincidunt, ligula in suscipit egestas, dui metus porta sem, eget pellentesque ligula elit id orci. Fusce viverra libero in velit iaculis, ut elementum lacus posuere. Phasellus et sollicitudin sem. Morbi nec enim vehicula felis iaculis pellentesque at nec tortor. Duis mollis, nibh non mattis porta, quam metus congue nisl, ut scelerisque ipsum lacus vel tortor. Quisque auctor, odio nec molestie placerat, nunc lacus pellentesque augue, eget faucibus odio justo eget nunc. Aenean tristique nunc neque, non placerat lorem egestas eu. Donec efficitur scelerisque dolor, eu tempor orci maximus a.

Background
Vestibulum non nunc eros. Aenean elementum metus dapibus, varius felis at, sollicitudin lorem. Aliquam erat volutpat. Sed eu enim nisl. Curabitur quis ligula urna. Nullam faucibus egestas justo, nec lobortis ipsum pellentesque vel. Phasellus volutpat malesuada dapibus. Vivamus gravida bibendum sapien nec sodales. Maecenas pulvinar condimentum enim ut consequat. Vivamus aliquet nec nunc at tempus. Nunc aliquam convallis efficitur. Proin erat orci, efficitur id pulvinar aliquet, fermentum non metus. Nunc sit amet tortor felis.

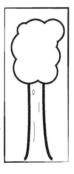

FIGURE 5.1   Example of a journal layout.

based on the 'research process', which is a recognisable sequence of stages that researchers follow when conducting a primary research study (see Figure 5.2). There are different perspectives on the number of fundamental stages, but at this point in your appraisal journey the most important things to know are what the key stages are and what order they occur in.

Familiarity with the research process will help you to read, understand, and appraise research papers, and you will see this term mentioned often in the upcoming chapters as we explain the various research designs and methods. A common term for the research article format is 'IMRaD'. This abbreviation stands for Introduction, Methods, Results, and Discussion and it is the reporting style that most journals present research in (Sollaci and Pereira 2004):

- **Introduction** presents the study context, for example what other research has been done on this topic, what is not yet understood about it, and why this research is needed.
- **Methods** presents the specific techniques used to recruit the participants and to gather and analyse the data needed to answer the research question.

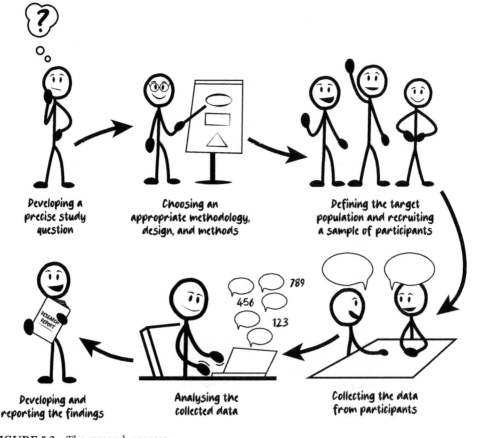

Developing a precise study question

Choosing an appropriate methodology, design, and methods

Defining the target population and recruiting a sample of participants

Developing and reporting the findings

Analysing the collected data

Collecting the data from participants

FIGURE 5.2   The research process.

- **Results** presents what was found from the collection and analysis of participants' data, in relation to the research question.
- **Discussion** presents how the study results fit within the wider evidence on the topic and suggests how the study results might be used.

It is useful to know about the IMRaD reporting style, because it can help you identify if you are reading a piece of research, rather than for example a reflection or discussion article. Although these may be useful evidence in some circumstances, they should not be appraised in the same way as research. However, knowing about IMRaD will not help you distinguish between primary and secondary research, the two main categories of research. Academic level 5 modules will generally require you to appraise a piece of primary research, because it introduces you to the foundational concepts of EBP, research evidence, and research appraisal.

While you are unlikely to be asked to appraise a piece of secondary research at academic level 5, bringing in secondary research as a contrast may enable you to give a more analytical explanation of primary research. If your assignment requires a discussion of evidence hierarchies or the implementation of research evidence in practice, then being able to explain the role of secondary research may be important.

 Research Essentials

Research process: a recognisable sequence of stages that researchers follow when conducting research. It begins with developing a precise research aim from the existing literature on the topic and continues through designing the study and its methods to analysing and reporting the findings.

IMRaD: a traditional research reporting format, which presents a research article in the order of introduction, methods, results, and discussion.

For this stage of your appraisal journey, the key thing is to be able to tell the difference between primary and secondary research. While primary research collects and analyses new data from participants, secondary research collects and analyses data from other previously conducted evidence. This is most often from existing primary research but can be other types of evidence. Therefore, secondary research is usually regarded as a stronger type of research than primary because its results are based on multiple pieces of evidence that may show agreement or a lack of consensus across a range of study findings. Secondary research is typically in the form of a literature review (for example a systematic review, narrative review, or scoping review) and generally aims to summarise what is known about a topic, what is not well understood, and what the overall quality of the existing evidence is. Secondary research in the context of evidence hierarchies is explained in Chapter 2, and in the context of evidence implementation and the different types of secondary research is explained in

TABLE 5.1   Is it primary or secondary research?

Article section	Primary research will generally have. . .	Secondary research will generally have. . .
Title/abstract	An active statement that the authors have conducted a **study**. For example, 'This study explored. . ..'	An active statement that the authors have conducted a **review**. For example, 'This review aimed to. . .'
Introduction	A description of what has been researched already on the topic, and what has not. The authors will explain how their study will go on to fill this gap in the evidence base.	An explanation of why it is necessary to summarise or synthesise all the current evidence on the subject under review. For example, because the best treatment or approach is not currently clear.
Research design	A description or statement of a specific study design. For example, a randomised controlled trial, a survey, or a qualitative design like ethnography.	A description of the review type or methodology. For example, a systematic literature review, narrative review, qualitative evidence synthesis, or systematic review.
Sample/ population	A description of the target population, how they were recruited, how many participants were included, and their characteristics. For example, their age, sex, occupation, severity of condition, etc.	No participants – instead a description of the amount and type of studies included will be given, as well as, sometimes, a matrix of all the final included studies.
Methods	A description of the data collection and analysis techniques used and how these were conducted. For example, questionnaires or interviews, statistical or thematic analysis.	A description of the search strategy used to gather the studies, what databases were used, and, sometimes, a flow chart showing how they filtered down to the final studies.

Chapter 10. Table 5.1 explains the core characteristics of primary and secondary research, as well as helping you to work out which type of research you are looking at.

The last suggestion for orientating yourself to research appraisal is locating the reporting guidelines for your type of study. Reporting guidelines are like checklists for research teams who are writing up their studies as articles to be published in journals. They were developed to ensure standardised and transparent reporting of research and they are available on the EQUATOR Network website (www.equator-network. org). The EQUATOR Network is an international organisation that evolved to address the problem of inconsistent and inadequate research reporting. The name stands for 'Enhancing the **QUA**lity and **T**ransparency **O**f health **R**esearch' and the website is a great source of information about study quality and robust research reporting generally. There are guidelines for randomised controlled trials, quantitative observational studies, and qualitative studies, as well as other types of research. Once you know what type of primary research you have, take a look at the relevant guidelines so that you have some ideas of the key issues that should have been reported in your study.

 Explore It

Go to the EQUATOR Network and take a look at all the different reporting guidelines. See what researchers should report in randomised control trials and qualitative research.

`www.equator-network.org`

5.3   GETTING TO GRIPS WITH YOUR PRIMARY STUDY

Now that you know you have a suitable primary study, it's beneficial to spend some time becoming familiar with the content in each of the sections in a general sense, before you start to work on the finer details of how it was conducted and what it found. At this stage, you should consider printing out your primary study and working from the physical rather than online version. There are advantages and disadvantages to working online and in print and ultimately it comes down to your personal preference, but there are a few things to think about.

Working entirely online is better for the environment of course! Online features can also be invaluable. For example, you can make as many notes as you like without the article becoming cluttered. You can also use the search function to find specific details within the article. For example, you may need information on the consent process and searching for 'consent' will take you straight there.

However, our experience suggests that when students print out their study they benefit in different ways. Making physical notes and highlighting is a different and more active way of interacting with the paper. It not only offers respite from screen work, but also enables a view of the study in its entirety, showing how the sections flow as part of the overall research process. So think about whether this method would be helpful for you. If you prefer to work purely online, it's advisable to use a larger device such as a laptop or good-sized tablet. Smaller screens and phones do not allow a clear overview and may make it tricky to see how the individual elements inform the study as a whole.

Whatever your preferred way of working, understanding what the different sections of the study present and where you can find key content can help you feel less anxious about starting your appraisal. Figure 5.3 illustrates the typical layout for a primary research article, while Table 5.2 explains what you are likely to find in each of the key sections.

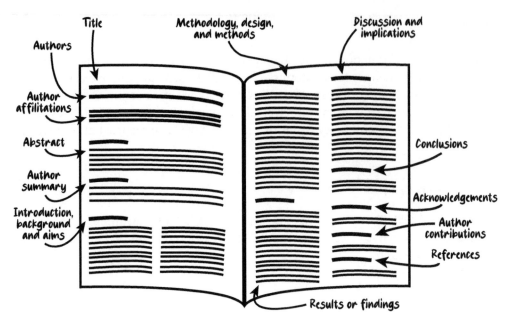

FIGURE 5.3 Typical layout of a published study.

TABLE 5.2 Typical content in a published research article.

Beginning	
Abstract	A concise summary of the entire paper and an excellent starting point for understanding the study as a whole.
Introduction	The introduction should explain the topic, key concepts, and why the study is necessary.
Background	There may be separate subheadings for a background or literature review, or this contextual information may be just in one introductory section.
Research question	It should lead to a clearly stated research aim or question, which is critical to an appraisal since the study is being evaluated on what it set out to answer This could take the form of an explicit hypothesis (a theory to be tested by the study) or an aim, possibly with several related objectives.
	NOTE: the research question is not the same as the article title. The title is worded so that the study can be searched for easily and may reflect the study design rather than the aim.
Middle	
Methodology	This is the overall approach to the research project and can be referred to in different ways (philosophy, beliefs and values, research paradigm) or not stated at all. Instead, it may be inferred by stating the study design For a primary study, it will be quantitative, qualitative, or mixed methods, and for appraisal it is crucial to identify this at an early stage.
Study design	This section reports the framework for how the study will be conducted and is more specific than the methodology It may not be headed or described as the 'study design', but may instead just be referred to by its name, for example 'This randomised controlled trial. . .' or 'This ethnographic design. . .'

TABLE 5.2 (Continued)

Methods	
Sampling and recruitment	This section should describe the population that the study is interested in (men over 65 with prostate cancer, for example) and the sample recruited to represent that population (men over 65 with prostate cancer attending a NHS hospital for medical follow-up appointments, for example). It should describe the methods used to select the sample, inclusion/exclusion criteria, how they were recruited, and the sample size
Data collection	This section should detail how the research team gathered the information they needed from participants. There may be one or more data collection methods, for example several questionnaires measuring different symptoms associated with arthritis (pain, fatigue, depression) or a combination of observation and interviews to explore patient experience.
Data analysis	This section should describe how the research team examined and interpreted the data collected from participants. Again, there could be one or multiple methods used.
Ethics	The location and detail of this section are variable. It typically states if ethical approval was obtained for the study and how consent was managed. There may also be detail on safeguarding and confidentiality issues, and conflicts of interest.
Results or findings	The researchers should describe the results of their analysis of the collected data, to answer their original research question. Depending on the methodology or design of the study, the findings may be presented numerically with tables or charts and some explanatory narrative, or it may be mainly narrative, with some participant quotes and supported by a table or model.
End	
Discussion	These sections may come as one or two sections or separated by subheadings. The discussion should give more interpretation of the findings, with reference to wider evidence on the topic. The researchers tend to bring in related research and existing guidelines or policies to demonstrate how their findings have contributed to understanding of the topic. The researchers should also acknowledge the limitations of their study and how they might have impacted on the findings.
Limitations	**NOTE**: The limitations section can be very helpful for your appraisal, but ensure that you do not just report what the research team reported.
Implications	Try to discuss using other sources and provide your own analysis. The implications section should make clear what the study findings can contribute to healthcare practice and how useful they can be in practical terms.
Conclusions	These are the take-home messages for the paper in relation to the original research question.
Acknowledgements	This section states who else supported the study, other than the authors.
References	Sources used to inform the article. **NOTE**: The references can be useful as a base to explore more about the study methods or findings.

Assignment Tip

Demonstrate that you know what primary research is and how it differs from other types of evidence. Try not to give just a definition or direct quote. Make your writing more analytical for academic writing at level 5 by contrasting primary against secondary research and noting how they differ in aim, characteristics, and strength of evidence for practice.

5.4   GATHER YOUR TOOLS

Now that you have a paper and can identify its main features, we suggest some supportive strategies that you can put in place now in order to make your research appraisal activities easier.

5.4.1   Research Resources

You've already got the best tool available for appraisal assignments in the form of this book! But what else might help you to understand and make effective critical points about research in your assignment?

A key source of support is your module reading list. These are typically now online and easily accessible for all and should cover the key areas that your module tutor wants you to focus on. Additionally, library staff will be able to help you find resources that are specific to your topic or field. Choosing a couple of core texts to develop and expand your general health research knowledge will be essential. There are many to choose from; try to view them online or on the library shelf to find one you feel comfortable with. There are also many journal articles that take you through research appraisal, and these will help to layer your work with different perspectives. See Box 5.1 for our top student choice recommendations.

Box 5.1   Student Choice Appraisal Resources

Aveyard, H. (2010). *Doing a Literature Review in Health and Social Care: A Practical Guide*. Maidenhead: McGraw-Hill Education.

Aveyard, H., and Sharp, P. (2013). *Beginner's Guide to Evidence-based Practice in Health and Social Care*. Milton Keynes: McGraw-Hill Education.

Burls, A. (2014). *What Is Critical Appraisal?* Newmarket: Hayward Medical Communications.

Gerrish, K., and Lathlean, J. (2015). *The Research Process in Nursing*, 7e. Hoboken, NJ: Wiley.

Greenhalgh, T. (2000). *How to Read a Paper: The Basics of Evidence Based Medicine*. London: Blackwell.

LoBiondo-Wood, G., and Haber, J. (2018). *Nursing Research: Methods and Critical Appraisal for Evidence-based Practice*, 9e (eds. G. LoBiondo-Wood and J. Haber). St Louis, MO: Elsevier.

Polit, D.F., and Beck, C.T. (2017). *Essentials of Nursing Research: Appraising Evidence for Nursing Practice*, 9e. Philadelphia: Lippincott Williams & Wilkins.

Walsh, M., and Wigens, L. (2003). *Introduction to Research*. Cheltenham: Nelson Thornes.

5.4.2   Peers and Group Support

While working on your own is necessarily the main way of developing your assignments, ensuring that you have some wider group support and periods of working collaboratively can be beneficial. Working with others is an opportunity to share your experiences, clarify areas of misunderstanding, and critically discuss your studies. Talking about your ideas allows you to articulate your thoughts in an informal way, which not only provides a break from reading and writing, but also stimulates critical thinking. Group work will expose you to the perspectives and research papers of others and this can be an enjoyable and easy way of learning about other research designs and methods. If your friend's study uses questionnaires to collect data and yours uses interviews, for example, you can discuss the strengths and limitations of both methods together and start to make notes on a point to include in your assignment. Contrasting different designs and methods not only demonstrates that you have a wide knowledge of research, but also makes writing more analytical and less descriptive.

Not everyone feels comfortable with group work. Some feel reluctant to share their ideas in case they are 'wrong'. But with appraisal, there often is no absolute right or wrong. Instead, the task is to weigh up possible strengths and limitations and these will vary depending on individual perspective and the research aim. Presenting these varying viewpoints in your assignment will demonstrate critical analysis, which is required to do well in level 5 assignments. So make the most of online discussion boards and class debate to pose questions, explore other perspectives, and test your ideas. Or, if you feel too uncomfortable, arrange for a small and perhaps familiar group to meet regularly throughout the module, as this will still allow for excellent peer support and critical discussion of each other's papers and ideas.

5.4.3   Make a Plan

Trying to appraise the whole study in one go can be overwhelming and unproductive, especially if anxiety has made you avoid it and you are close to the deadline. Trying to do too much at once can lead to unfocused skimming through books and websites, as well as directionless writing that is unlikely to produce a good-quality assignment.

Luckily, the fact that research follows a standard sequence of steps means that appraisal assignments can be easily broken down into more manageable chunks. Developing a study plan that capitalises on this helps you to work in a more efficient and methodical way. For example, using the sections of Table 5.2 you might plan to *identify* all the key elements of your study in the early part of your module, before moving on to *appraise* these elements as you progress, and in the later stages adapting your notes into paragraphs.

Working in these focused blocks can be much more efficient than reading about lots of unrelated aspects and creating too many disconnected notes. Advanced planning also allows you to make the most of your available study time. Even if you only have a couple of hours free for study before work or collecting children from school, you can focus in on one element and make visible progress. For example, in two hours you could read about and write notes on just the design of your study. This would enable you to have the foundations of an appraisal point for your study design and to clarify your understanding with your tutor at your next contact time. This reduces anxiety and leaves more energy for learning.

5.5   WRITING ABOUT THE TYPE OF RESEARCH AND ITS LAYOUT IN YOUR ASSIGNMENT

Establishing if your research is primary or secondary is important and for the purposes of appraisal you should demonstrate that you know what primary research is, how it is different to other types of research, and the general quality markers related to it (these will be covered in Chapters 7 and 8). It may also be pertinent to discuss if the research article has missed key details of the study. Using the appropriate reporting guidelines (see Section 5.2 earlier), you may be able to argue that the steps of the analysis process have not been described sufficiently for thorough appraisal, for instance. You would need to add what should have been reported and why that was important for the appraisal, but this type of point still enables you to demonstrate your knowledge of research quality. See the examples that follow for how to discuss primary and secondary research in assignments.

Issues relating to journal layout and style should not generally be included in your appraisal assignment. While they may make a difference to your ability to read a study and understand it, layout and style issues reflect journal formatting requirements and not the quality of the research or the applicability of its findings. Therefore, spend your word count discussing more important issues.

5.6   ASSIGNMENT EXAMPLES

Example 1: Both of these studies are primary research. Primary research refers to studies where researchers generate and analyse their own data (Bermingham 2020a). Secondary research refers to the analysis of primary research by collecting together and reviewing various pieces of primary research (Bermingham 2020b). Thus, it could be argued that secondary research is more reliable than primary research. Therefore, having research from both approaches is useful when considering impact on practice.

Example 2: There are some limitations to primary sources of research however. For example, small sample sizes and specificity of settings mean that they are not necessarily reliable to generalise from, nor do they always provide a conclusive answer (Topping 2015). Therefore, primary studies alone provide insufficient evidence to inform clinical practice. Practitioners should instead seek a more extensive overview of relevant research in order to provide the most appropriate, evidence-based interventions (Gerrish 2015).

Example 3: Secondary research can comprehensively summarise relevant evidence (Beecroft et al. 2015), often collecting and appraising large volumes of data to assess the strength and quality of multiple study findings. They also allow for quicker assimilation of vast amounts of information and facilitating the implementation of EBP. On the topic of compression bandaging, a meta-analysis by O'Meara et al. (2012) identified compression stockings as a viable alternative to multi-layer bandages, highlighting equal clinical efficacy, improved patient acceptance and cost-effectiveness.

5.7   END-OF-CHAPTER CHECKPOINT

		Comment/ notes
I can explain the difference between primary and secondary research	Yes/no	
I have chosen/been given a research paper for appraisal. I have identified that it is appropriate for my assignment	Yes/no	
I know what the IMRaD structure of a research paper is	Yes/no	
I can list the stages of the research process in the correct order	Yes/no	
I can explain briefly what each step in the research process requires	Yes/no	
I have accessed the reading list for my research module and chosen some core texts and journal articles	Yes/no	
I have explored opportunities for group work with my peer group or tutor	Yes/no	
I have printed and read though my whole research paper	Yes/no	

		Comment/ notes
I feel ready to start planning my assignment	Yes/no	
On a scale of 1–5, how confident do you feel about the content in this chapter?		

5.8   CHAPTER SUMMARY

In this chapter we have explained that it is common to feel overwhelmed and anxious about appraising a research study for an assignment. We suggested that this is related to a lack of familiarity with different types of research, how research is reported, and how research is conducted. A range of strategies and tips have been suggested, and these are based on gradually building your familiarity with research reporting, its key elements and features, so that your research paper itself feels clearer to work from.

We also advised making time to gather helpful resources such as relevant reading, discussion opportunities, and a study planner. Having used the end-of-chapter checklist you should now be able to see if you need to clarify any aspects, or if you are ready to move on to learning about research methods and appraisal in more depth.

REFERENCES

Beecroft, C., Booth, A., and Rees, A. (2015). Finding the evidence. In: *The Research Process in Nursing*, 7e (ed. K. Gerrish and J. Lathlean), 89–104. Chichester: Wiley Blackwell.

Bermingham, R. (2020a). Study designs: Primary research. *POST*. https://post.parliament.uk/study-designs-secondary-research (accessed 4 December 2023).

Bermingham, R. (2020b). Study designs: Secondary research. *POST*. https://post.parliament.uk/study-designs-primary-research (accessed 4 December 2023).

Earley, M.A. (2014). A synthesis of the literature on research methods education. *Teaching in Higher Education* 19 (3): 242–253. https://doi.org/10.1080/13562517.2013.860105.

Gerrish, K. (2015). Research and development in nursing. In: *Research Process in Nursing*, 7e (ed. K. Gerrish and J. Lathlean), 3–13. Chichester: Wiley Blackwell.

O'Meara, S., Cullum, N., Nelson, E.A., and Dumville, J.C. (2012). Compression for venous leg ulcers. *Cochrane Database of Systematic Reviews* 11 (11), CD000265. https://doi.org/10.1002/14651858.CD000265.pub3.

Papanastasiou, E.C. and Zembylas, M. (2008). Anxiety in undergraduate research methods courses: its nature and implications. *International Journal of Research and Method in Education* 31 (2): 155–167. https://doi.org/10.1080/17437270802124616.

Ramsay, A., Wicking, K., and Yates, K. (2020). In what ways does online teaching create a positive attitude towards research in nursing students studying a first year evidence-based practice undergraduate subject online? *Nurse Education in Practice* 44: 102744. https://doi.org/10.1016/j.nepr.2020.102744.

Sollaci, L.B. and Pereira, M.G. (2004). The introduction, methods, results, and discussion (IMRAD) structure: a fifty-year survey. *Journal of the Medical Library Association* 92 (3): 364–371.

Topping, A. (2015). The quantitative-qualitative continuum. In: *Research Process in Nursing*, 7e (ed. K. Gerrish and J. Lathlean), 159–171. Chichester: Wiley Blackwell.

PART II

DIGGING IN THE DETAIL!

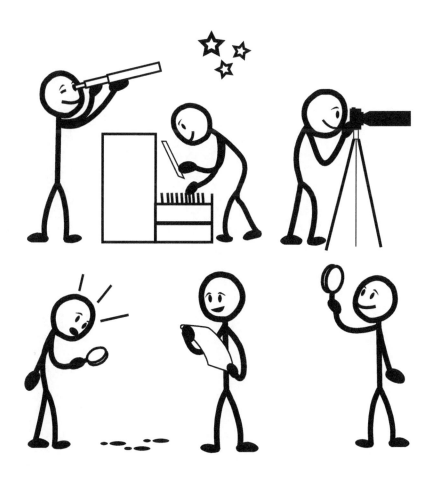

CHAPTER 6

Critical Appraisal

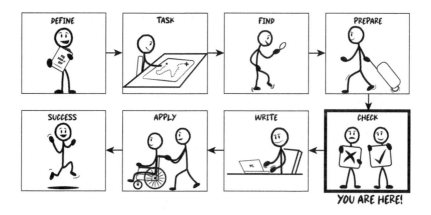

FIVE THINGS TO LEARN FROM THIS CHAPTER

1. It is imperative to correctly identify your chosen research paper as quantitative, qualitative, or mixed methods *before* embarking on critical appraisal.

2. Quantitative researchers like control, standardisation, measurement, and objectivity.

3. Qualitative researchers like naturally occurring events, making sense of the world, unique experiences, and subjectivity; and mixed-methods researchers like being pragmatic and doing 'what works' to answer their research question.

Critical Appraisal Skills for Healthcare Students: A Practical Guide to Writing Evidence-based Practice Assignments, First Edition. Charlotte J. Whiffin, Donna Barnes, and Lorraine Henshaw.
© 2024 John Wiley & Sons Ltd. Published 2024 by John Wiley & Sons Ltd.

4. You need to be able to correctly identify the research design used in the study and ask specific appraisal questions relevant to this research type.

5. Critical appraisal is a systematic process of assessing the quality of the research, whether we can trust the results, and whether the results are relevant to practice.

FIVE MINUTES WITH TOM, RADIOGRAPHY STUDENT

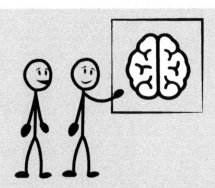

Was there anything you enjoyed about appraising research?
I enjoyed appraising research, and it has helped me to further understand the importance of research within my daily practice and in a wider scale.

What did you find hardest about appraising your paper?
I was initially worried about appraising research, especially having to compare qualitative (my chosen study) to quantitative study, which I did not feel as confident about. It can be hard to work out the details of the study initially. I had one study; I knew it was a questionnaire method, but I could not tell if it was quantitative or qualitative. It seemed to have elements of both, but it did not report clearly its methodology or design. So sometimes it takes a while to work that out before you can even get going on the appraisal.

What strategies helped you to complete your appraisal?
Break it down into small elements – whether that is the stages of the research process, or for a dissertation, the different chapters and subheadings. Work on each one at a time so you can focus your reading around the issues.

Also, use an appraisal tool like CASP and distinguish between factual evidence and opinions to determine applicability. Once you learn the skills it all makes sense.

What advice do you have for anyone appraising research?
Use the available tools to help you. CASP has the tools for both qualitative and quantitative research that will help you find the information you need to appraise the research effectively. I used

the CASP tool to thoroughly appraise the articles I used for my dissertation. I ensured I answered all the questions and gathered all the information required. This will give you a full insight into the paper.

6.1   INTRODUCTION

If you have worked your way through Part 1 of this textbook, you should now have:

- A research paper or papers to appraise.
- A broad overview of what the study is about, how it was conducted, and what it found.
- A clear understanding of the assessment criteria for your assignment and insight into how to achieve these.

In Part 2 of this textbook, we will look in more detail at the methods and techniques used by the researchers to conduct their study, whether these methods and techniques affect the quality of the study in any way, and therefore whether we should trust what the researchers found. We will introduce you to the 'EDECA' model for appraisal, which will unpick key points in the 'Ethics, Design, Enrol, Collect, and Analysis' sections of published research (Chapters 7 and 8). We will then show you how to write about these points in an assignment (Chapter 9) and, lastly, we look at implementing evidence into practice (Chapter 10).

6.2   HOW TO USE PART 2

To work through Part 2, you will need to know what type of research you are appraising. Once you have decided which type it is, you can then move to the relevant section of this book to appraise the research. But how do you know what type of study you have?

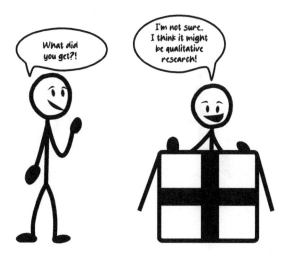

We will now briefly introduce you to each of these methodologies. You may find that you naturally prefer one over another. You may not understand why at this stage: one just seems to suit the way you see the world, the way you think about problems and their solutions, the way you practise, the way you behave. There is a reason for this, but for now we will concentrate on the core characteristics of qualitative, quantitative, and mixed-methods research so you can easily identify each type of study. However, remember that all rules are meant to be broken, so the characteristics listed here should be seen as *often* the case, rather than *always* true.

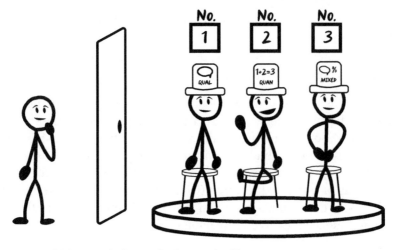

Who will it be: quantitative, qualitative, or mixed?

6.3   INTRODUCING THE QUANTITATIVE RESEARCHER

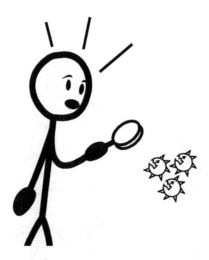

Likes	Dislikes
The scientific approach	Outside influence
Control	Things that cannot be measured
Standardisation	Spontaneity
Reason and logic	Lack of advanced planning
Rules	Unplanned change
Pre-determined methods	Lack of control
Measurement	
Objectivity	
Experiments	

Meet your quantitative researcher. They would most likely say they follow the 'scientific method'. They are interested in measurement, statistics, cause and effect; they like to be in control of their research and plan meticulously for all eventualities. Quantitative researchers are particularly interested in how the world can be explained through quantification and standardised measures.

The quantitative researcher loves to explore cause and effect by conducting experiments where they can study what happens when they change something, for example a treatment or method (these 'somethings' are called variables), and measure the response (the outcome). Quantitative researchers examine the outcome of their experiments numerically and describe the relationships they think may exist between what happened after (the effect) with what happened before (the cause).

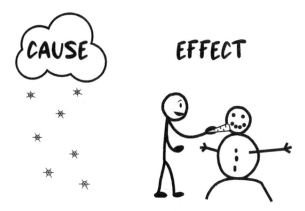

In health research this is often through experiments called randomised controlled trials (RCTs), where one group of people gets treatment A and another gets treatment B. The researchers try to ensure that the groups getting the different treatments are the same at the start of the trial, i.e. the same in terms of age, sex, severity of illness, but the individual allocation to the group is random. Therefore, if the groups are different in any way after the trial, the researchers can assume that the reason for the difference is the different treatments. There are of course lots of other things going on in studies like these (called confounding factors), but researchers try to reduce the impact of these on their trial to increase their confidence in the results. Researchers use statistical tests to find out if the differences between the groups could have happened by chance or if there is an actual difference and the results support their hypothesis (the thing they are trying to prove). If the likelihood of the result occurring by chance is low (as determined by the statistical test), the researchers can be confident that there is a real difference in treatment response between the groups, supporting their hypothesis, and that they can expect this treatment response in other people outside of those who took part in their study.

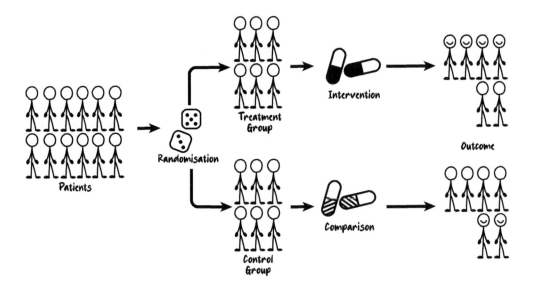

So if you like being in control, experimenting with new ideas, testing out your ideas, and using quantification, measurement, and statistics to determine the answers to questions, you are most likely attracted to quantitative research.

In a research paper you can identify a quantitative study by:

- The heavy reliance on numerical representation of the data, in the form of tables, graphs, and mathematical calculations.
- A stated 'hypothesis' or specific research aim of quantifying something, or measuring its effect on something else.
- Terms such as variables, primary outcomes, or statistical tests.

6.4   INTRODUCING THE QUALITATIVE RESEARCHER

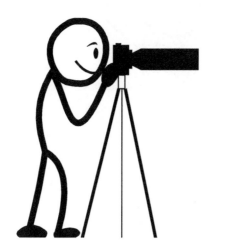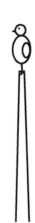

Likes	Dislikes
Observing the naturally occurring world	Control and manipulation
Social science	Treating everyone the same
Subjectivity and getting close to the participants	Distance from participants
Immersing themselves in the issue under investigation	Reducing or simplifying complex issues
Understanding the 'inside' perspective	Intervening in naturally occurring events
New and complex problems	A superficial understanding of a problem
Exploring experiences and perceptions and different views	Inflexibility

Meet your typical qualitative researcher. They are most likely to be found in the social sciences working with participants and getting to understand their stories. They are interested in what people think, how they behave, and how they are different from each other. Qualitative researchers like to find out about things we do not know a lot about yet, to shine light on new problems and in new ways, to help people understand the worlds of those who are affected. When something is poorly understood, qualitative research is a very effective research method to find out more about it.

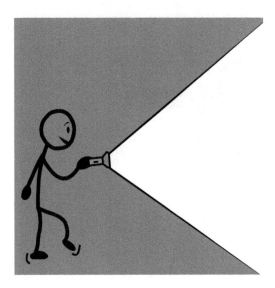

The field of qualitative research developed from a need to investigate health issues in a different way than was possible with quantitative research. After all, numbers are never enough to understand the world we live in and our experience of living in it. Albert Einstein captured this sentiment well.

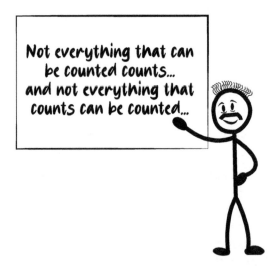

The topic that qualitative researchers are investigating is often called the 'phenomenon' and researchers want to know what this phenomenon is like from the perspective of a particular population, group, or culture. Qualitative researchers may also interpret experiences people have and the personal meanings they attach to them. They may see these experiences from different perspectives like gender or race and create new theories about social processes or culture where they do not yet exist.

The qualitative researcher needs methods that enable them to develop insight, rich description, and authentic representation of participant data.

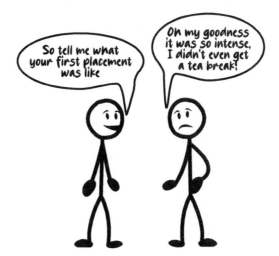

So if you like exploring problems from the inside out, if you value different viewpoints and want to understand why these different views exist, if you want to explore experiences and understand their meaning, you are most likely attracted to qualitative research.

In a research paper you can usually identify qualitative research by:

- A research aim that is focused on exploring the experiences or perceptions of people or groups.
- Terms such as phenomena, theory, themes, or insider perspective.
- A reliance on direct quotes to help readers understand the findings.

6.5   INTRODUCING THE MIXED-METHODS RESEARCHER

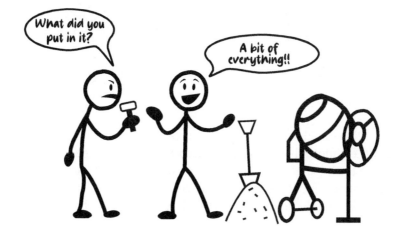

Likes	Dislikes
Complex research questions	Having to choose between methods
Measuring and exploring the issue at hand	Rules
Choice	Restrictions
Being pragmatic	Paradigm wars
Doing what works	

Mixed-methods researchers are usually found researching complex health and social care problems where a restriction to using only quantitative or qualitative methods would not allow them to answer their research question in full. It is because of this that they usually think in a pragmatic way about combining different methods and use the principle of 'what works best' rather than being restricted to choosing subjective *or* objective methods. However, what you should be able to tell from the introductions to quantitative and qualitative researchers is that these people like very different things, in fact most of their likes and dislikes are diametrically opposed, so bringing these two contrasting views together can be quite difficult.

Think for a minute about different political viewpoints, one far right and one far left. These people find it hard to work naturally together because of their contrasting belief systems. In research, opposing views of how knowledge is constructed led to years of what was known as the 'paradigm wars'. OK, they were not exactly a 'war', but this metaphor represented the conflict between quantitative and qualitative researchers about which way is better to conduct research.

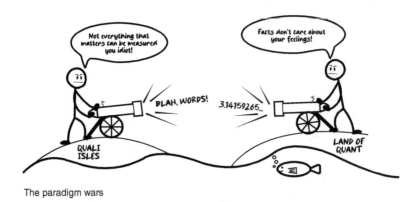

The paradigm wars

So, if you like the idea of 'having your cake and eating it' and are not concerned too much by the philosophical reasons underpinning knowledge generation, you may be attracted to this type of research. Research papers using mixed methods will normally have results from statistical calculations *and* findings using direct quotes or similar. In an ideal world the researcher will identify their study as mixed methods in the title and/or abstract.

For some people 'a bit of everything' may feel like the perfect solution, but here are a few words of caution:

- A qualitative study may report some quantitative data without the study being classed as mixed methods.
- A quantitative study may report on some open-ended survey responses without the study being classed as mixed methods.
- To appraise a mixed-methods study you need to understand *both* quantitative and qualitative principles *and* how they are able to exist within the same study. So it is much harder!

It is because of these problems that most commonly our advice to students is to appraise a paper that is quite clearly *either* quantitative *or* qualitative until they are confident about these primary research designs. If on the other hand you are required to review an evidence base rather than select one or two papers, mixed methods may be unavoidable and as such we have included some discussion of mixed methods in this book. The following chapters cover quantitative and qualitative approaches in some detail and if you do have a mixed-methods research article, you will need to use the relevant sections of these chapters on each of the research methods to appraise these approaches individually. You should then refer to our Key Fact Sheet for Mixed-Methods Research (found in the Appendix) to appraise how the researchers have 'mixed the methods'. This fact sheet also includes some really useful additional resources.

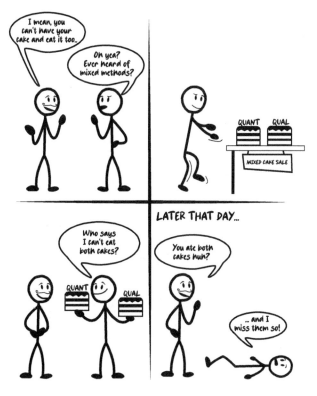

6.6   DECISION TIME

If you are still not sure what type of research you have, answer the questions in Table 6.1 and then use the decision tool in Figure 6.1.

6.7   THE FINAL DECISION

To appraise a paper properly you should ask questions that relate directly to the methods used. While you can appraise based on generic qualitative or quantitative questions, it is far better to judge if the methods used were employed in the correct way for the type of qualitative or quantitative research being carried out. See Table 6.2 for some examples of specific research designs relating to qualitative and quantitative methodology.

In an ideal world, if the paper has been written and reported properly the research design should be reported in the title or abstract. Unfortunately, this is not always the case. Where the design is clearly reported you can be confident of what type of study

TABLE 6.1   Questions to identify methodology.

	A	B
At the beginning		
Introduction	Talks about the importance of individual experiences. The subject area is underexplored or not well understood.	Clearly defines the people, the specific 'thing' of interest (e.g. an intervention), and what they expect to find out.
Research aim/ question	Exploratory	Explanatory ± hypothesis
In the middle		
Researchers use...	Interviews, observations, diaries.	Questionnaires or defined measures such as weight, height, blood pressure, pain score.
Analysis is performed using...	Qualitative analysis, e.g. thematic, content, narrative, grounded theory and phenomenological approaches.	Statistical tests, e.g. T tests, Chi squared, ANOVA, averages, standard deviation.
At the end		
Results are presented as...	Themes, subthemes, stories, theory.	Numerical results from the statistical tests used (e.g. p = 0.05; OR = 0.2–1.6)
Results look like...	Lots of direct quotes	Tables, charts, graphs, P values, confidence intervals.

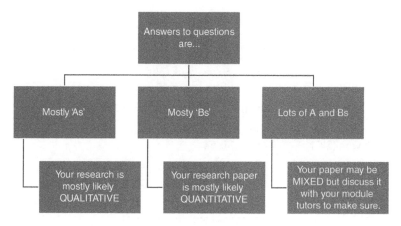

FIGURE 6.1   Research methodology decision tool.

TABLE 6.2   Specific research designs.

Qualitative research designs	Quantitative research designs	Mixed methods
Phenomenology	Randomised controlled trial	Mixed
Narrative	Quasi-experimental	
Ethnography	Cohort	
Grounded theory	Case–control	
Case study	Survey	

you have. If it is not, you can use a generic appraisal tool. However, to progress in this book you may want to check with a module tutor before committing to an appraisal tool for a specific research design.

Aim: To correctly identify your paper.

Instructions: Complete a similar table to the one below for your chosen research paper.

Author, year, country	Jones et al. (2022), USA
Research title	Efficacy of talking therapies in school-aged children
My paper is. . .	Quantitative
The research design used is. . .	A randomised controlled trial

6.8   PREPARING FOR APPRAISAL

To prepare for a critical appraisal task you need to decide on a tool, or framework, to help guide you through this process. Critical appraisal tools use a checklist approach to evaluate evidence (Buccheri and Sharifi 2017). Table 6.3 provides some recommended

TABLE 6.3   Recommended resources for appraisal.

Organisation	Website
Critical Appraisal Skills Programme (CASP)	`https://casp-uk.net`
Joanna Briggs Institute (JBI)	`https://jbi.global/critical-appraisal-tools`
Scottish Intercollegiate Guidelines Network (SIGN)	`www.sign.ac.uk/what-we-do/methodology/checklists`
BMJ	`https://bestpractice.bmj.com/info/toolkit/ebm-toolbox/critical-appraisal-checklists`
Centre for Evidence-Based Medicine	`https://www.cebm.ox.ac.uk/resources/ebm-tools/critical-appraisal-tool`

critical appraisal tools; however, there are many more. In fact, Katrak et al. (2004) found 121 published critical appraisal tools. With no 'one size fits all' or 'gold standard' tool that all healthcare professionals should use, this can make choosing the right tool for the job somewhat difficult (Buccheri and Sharifi 2017). Furthermore, the language of research is often seen as inaccessible (Rebar and Macnee 2010), and given that these tools are often written in a similar way this creates a significant barrier to their use.

Therefore, in Chapters 7 and 8 of this book we will show you our own way to appraise the research designs listed in Table 6.2. If you have a study design not listed here, you may want to look for another textbook or appraisal tool to help guide you through the appraisal task.

 Assignment Tip

Whatever type of study you are appraising, consider demonstrating that you know about the other type. For example, if you are appraising a qualitative study, you could explain its core characteristics and then contrast these with those of quantitative research or vice versa. Alternatively, you could suggest how a quantitative study might have researched the topic differently, e.g. measuring the effectiveness of a current treatment rather than exploring the experience of living with the condition. As you are being assessed on your understanding of research and EBP, showing that you have knowledge of both may strengthen your assignment.

6.9   FOCUSING IN ON APPRAISAL

It is true that there are more facets to appraisal than we will provide in this textbook. However, given that the focus of this text is level 5 assignments, and the undergraduate students writing them, we want you to be able to focus on a limited number of key points and core principles when reading primary research. We will nevertheless signpost you to more advanced concepts where appropriate should you want to further your understanding beyond those covered here.

At the end of this chapter, you can navigate to the quantitative (Chapter 7) or qualitative (Chapter 8) chapter of this book, depending on the methodology of the study you are appraising. In these chapters, we will explain the key principles and quality issues of each methodology. Subsequently, we provide you with a Key Facts Sheet relating to several different designs. This will summarise the important characteristics of each design and their common aim(s). We will cite some examples of real studies that use this design that you can review in your own time and then present three unique design issues. The fact sheets then move on to our 'EDECA' appraisal considerations (Ethics, Design, Enrol, Collect, Analyse) and what you need to look out for in these types of studies. Finally, each Key Facts Sheet finishes with a mini glossary and key resources to advance your understanding.

Once you have got to grips with the design and methods of your study, Chapter 9 will help you to turn your critical ideas into analytical writing suitable for an academic level 5 assignment. It will give you some practical strategies in the form of a tool to break down a research study into manageable elements and construct meaningful points about its quality.

However, before we move on to doing the appraisal, we need to set the scene for what critical appraisal is and why it is relevant to you as a registered professional.

6.10 CRITICAL APPRAISAL

Critical appraisal helps you to carefully, and systematically, consider the strengths and weaknesses of the research paper and make a judgement about whether the study can be applied to clinical practice (Whiffin and Hasselder 2013; Burls 2014). The outcome of appraisal should be about how much confidence you have in the findings. If you are over- or under-critical, you may not interpret or apply the result of the study appropriately (Tod et al. 2022).

Now you are familiar with the elements involved in critical appraisal, it is time to introduce some explicit definitions. These may come in handy for your assignment!

Critical appraisal is. . .

> . . .*the process of carefully and systematically examining research to judge its trustworthiness, and its value and relevance in a particular context.* (Burls 2014, p. 1)

> . . .*the structured process of examining a piece of evidence in order to determine its strengths and limitations and therefore the relevance or weight it should have in addressing your research question/argument.* (Aveyard and Sharp 2017 p. 138)

The systematic, unbiased, careful examination of each aspect of studies to judge their strengths, limitations, trustworthiness, meaning and applicability to practice. (Grove et al. 2016, p. 432)

 Assignment Tip

Definitions are often necessary to include in your assignment, e.g. the definition of critical appraisal. However, do not use too many and make sure you know why you picked the one you did, as some are better than others!

 Aim: To improve your understanding of the definitions of critical appraisal

Instructions: Review the definitions of critical appraisal provided in this chapter. What are the similarities and differences you can see in them?

In a 2011 Cochrane review of teaching critical appraisal skills in healthcare settings by Horsley et al. (2011), the following, more dated, definition from Last (1988) was used:

> *The process of assessing and interpreting evidence (usually published research) by systematically considering its validity (closeness to the truth), results and relevance to the individual's work.* (Last 1988, cited in Horsley et al. 2011)

Given the role of Cochrane within evidence-based practice (as outlined in Chapter 2), we felt that this definition warranted inclusion in this book as the 'go-to' definition for the following reasons:

- The definition makes it clear that critical appraisal is a 'process', which suggests that you are actively doing something.
- Using the word 'interpretation' tells us there are judgements being made and that it is up to you to assess the research and the value of the findings rather than just accept them.
- The word 'systematically' is important because it reaffirms the need to evaluate the paper according to a fixed framework.
- There is the interesting inclusion of 'closeness to the truth', which refers to the accuracy of the methods applied and whether we can trust in the findings.
- Finally, there is reference to 'relevance' in this definition. This is important because the research could be very well conducted but have no application to

the population the clinician is working with, and therefore there must be some evaluation of the use of the research within the context of your own professional practice.

Checkpoint Activity

Aim: To record your preferred definition of critical appraisal.

Instructions: Having read all the definitions of critical appraisal provided in this book, which definition do you prefer and why? Make a note of this definition here and the reference for it so that you can cite in your assignment if required.

_____

_____

_____

_____

6.11   WHAT DOES BEING 'CRITICAL' MEAN?

It easy to think that being 'critical' means picking fault (Duffy et al. 2009). In fact, some students can feel quite deflated when they can find little wrong with their chosen study because they feel they have nothing to write about for their assignment! Students may then try to find what they think is a 'bad' study to critically appraise instead.

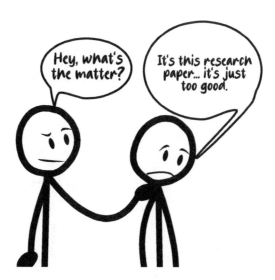

Our advice is, rather than searching for something that may be more substantially flawed, you can still use the 'good' paper for your assignment because critical appraisal is not about 'criticising' a paper for all its faults. Critical appraisal is a process of questioning, assessing, and judging. It is the process of being critical that is of value here and not what the process leads to – judging the paper as good or bad.

In reality, research is rarely judged in this way anyway. Even good studies have limitations and bad studies may still have some merit, so your job is to evaluate the impact of these merits and limitations on the potential value of the research to practice. So be assured that you can use any quality of research for your assignment. It's what you do with it that matters!

Now you understand that 'critical' is not a synonym for 'criticise', we can unpack the skill of criticality a bit further. Criticality is the foundation of critical thinking, which is a key attribute of professional practice (Sharples et al. 2017). So developing your skills of critical thinking will contribute to your development in practice as a healthcare professional.

Critical thinking involves (Facione 1990; Sharples et al. 2017):

- The cognitive skills of interpretation, analysis, evaluation, inference, explanation, and self-regulation.
- An approach to life in general that is inquisitive, well informed, flexible, and open minded.
- An ordered, diligent, reasoned, persistent, and precision approach to specific questions or problems.

Remember that critical appraisal is a balanced assessment of strengths and weaknesses, including the ethical, financial, legal, and pragmatic decisions made by researchers.

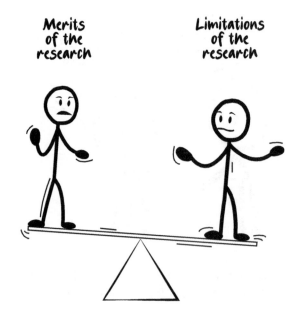

Merits of the research

Limitations of the research

6.12   'AM I DOING IT RIGHT?'

In our experience students often want to know they are doing appraisal 'right'. However, appraisal is an interpretative process and will be influenced by the reviewer's personal, theoretical, and gendered experience (Tod et al. 2022). Add to this your different professional experiences and practice contexts. This then leads to different appraisers reaching different conclusions. Since different views are to be expected, rather than asking if you are 'doing it right', think more about what is leading you to have the views you do and the conclusions you have reached. This is an important part of critical thinking, which is key to critical appraisal.

 Assignment Tip

You can demonstrate your understanding of critical appraisal in your assignment by writing about why it is important and what it involves.

6.13   WRITING ABOUT CRITICAL APPRAISAL IN YOUR ASSIGNMENT

As we have said before (and will continue to emphasise through the rest of the book!), the key to writing about important module concepts well is to *analyse* rather than *describe*. We discuss this in more depth and in relation to appraising the different elements of your study in Chapter 9. In terms of the concept of appraisal, it is important to show a comprehensive understanding of its meaning, its role within the EBP process, and why it is an important skill to develop as a registered professional.

To do this well, it is worth spending time reading about it in a few different health research resources and discussing the differences in definitions or guidance for how to conduct a good appraisal. Using a single source makes it difficult to be analytical, as you are more likely to state what a single author says about appraisal. However, when you use a range of sources it gives you the opportunity to note similarities and differences in how the concept is understood, how it has evolved over time, or how it is applied differently across various fields or professions. See the student examples that follow and make use of the activities in this chapter to craft an analytical explanation of appraisal.

6.14   ASSIGNMENT EXAMPLES

Example 1: This assignment critically appraises a piece of primary research by Kuo et al. (2020), by working through the five stages of the EBP cycle and focusing particularly on the stages of appraisal and application. Jolley (2013) describes research as systematically obtaining and analysing data to answer a specific question. It is vital to determine the quality of research however and critical appraisal is used to facilitate that, by identifying its strengths and weaknesses to conclude its significance before applying the findings for EBP (Gerrish and Lathlean 2015).

Example 2: The use of EBP is important for health professionals. It is a professional requirement that research and evidence should inform practice (NMC 2018) and that health professionals must be able to demonstrate EBP skills, using their knowledge and experience to make evidence-based decisions and to solve problems (NMC 2018). Being able to appraise research is a key part of EBP and it helps establish whether research is reliable and trustworthy, as well as its value and relevance to one's own practice (Morrison 2023).

Example 3: It is essential to ensure that research, which is a type of evidence that systematically gathers data for a specific question, goes through rigorous research appraisal before it is applied (Department of Health 2005). Critically evaluating the quality of evidence, taking into consideration its strengths and limitations, will demonstrate the robustness of a study (Raby and McNaughton 2021). This process will support the development of EBP skills for health professionals as well as showing if the study findings are applicable to the health professional's practice (Tod et al. 2022).

Example 4: The Critical Appraisal Skills Programme (CASP) appraisal tools for qualitative and RCT studies (CASP 2020) will support this evaluation of primary research. Critical appraisal tools can help distinguish between strong and weak evidence (Tod et al. 2022) and the process of conducting a critical appraisal can enhances nurses' skills to determine whether research is credible and relevant to their patients (Al-Jundi 2017). Long et al. (2020) acknowledge CASP's strengths but suggest it is a generic tool for novice researchers. Nevertheless, Dalton et al. (2017) demonstrate how CASP is the most widely used for appraisal in health related studies due to its quality of measuring research standards.

6.15   END-OF-CHAPTER CHECKPOINT

		Comment/notes
I know what type of research I am going to appraise	Yes/no	Quantitative, qualitative, or mixed?
I can identify the main characteristics of quantitative research	Yes/no	
I can identify the main characteristics of qualitative research	Yes/no	
I can identify the main characteristics of mixed-methods research	Yes/no	

		Comment/notes
I know where to obtain the appropriate critical appraisal checklist	Yes/no	
I can provide a definition for critical appraisal	Yes/no	
I have strategies to help me manage the critical appraisal process	Yes/no	
On a scale of 1–5, how confident do you feel about the content in this chapter?		

6.16 CHAPTER SUMMARY

In this chapter you have been introduced to the different types of research and their core commitments. We have explained how to identify research as quantitative, qualitative, and mixed methods and you should now be able to determine what type of study you are going to appraise. We have also explored the basic principles of critical appraisal, its definition, and its relevance to professional practice. You should now be all set for the detailed appraisal work in the next two chapters.

REFERENCES

Al-Jundi, A. (2017). Critical appraisal of clinical research. *Journal of Clinical and Diagnostic Research* https://doi.org/10.7860/jcdr/2017/26047.9942.

Aveyard, H. and Sharp, P. (2017). *A Beginners Guide to Evidence Based Practice in Health and Social Care*. Maidenhead: McGraw-Hill Education.

Buccheri, R.K. and Sharifi, C. (2017). Critical appraisal tools and reporting guidelines for evidence-based practice. *Worldviews on Evidence-Based Nursing* 14 (6): 463–472.

Burls, A. (2014). *What Is Critical Appraisal? Newmarket*. Hayward Medical Communications.

Critical Appraisal Skills Programme (CASP) (2020). CASP checklists. https://casp-uk.net/casp-tools-checklists (accessed 4 December 2023).

Dalton, J., Booth, A., Noyes, J., and Sowden, A.J. (2017). Potential value of systematic reviews of qualitative evidence in informing user-centered health and social care: findings from a descriptive overview. *Journal of Clinical Epidemiology* 88: 37–46.

Department of Health (2005). *Research Governance Framework for Health and Social Care*, 2e. London: Department of Health.

Duffy, K., Hastie, E., McCallum, J. et al. (2009). Academic writing: using literature to demonstrate critical analysis. *Nursing Standard* 23 (47): 35–40.

Facione, P. (1990). Critical thinking: A statement of expert consensus for purposes of educational assessment and instruction (The Delphi Report). Newark, DE: American Philosophical Association. https://eric.ed.gov/?id=ED315423 (accessed 4 December 2023).

Gerrish, K. and Lathlean, J. (2015). *Research Process in Nursing*. Chichester: Wiley Blackwell.

Grove, S.K., Burns, N., and Gray, J. (2016). *The Practice of Nursing Research Appraisal, Synthesis, and Generation of Evidence*, 8e. New York: Elsevier.

Horsley, T., Hyde, C., Santesso, N. et al. (2011). Teaching critical appraisal skills in healthcare settings. *Cochrane Database of Systematic Reviews* (11): CD001270.

Jolley, J. (2013). *Introducing Research and Evidence-based Practice for Nursing and Healthcare Professionals*. Abingdon: Routledge.

Katrak, P., Bialocerkowski, A.E., Massy-Westropp, N. et al. (2004). A systematic review of the content of critical appraisal tools. *BMC Medical Research Methodology* 4 (1): 1–11.

Kuo, S.Y., Wu, J.C., Chen, H.W. et al. (2020). Comparison of the effects of simulation training and problem-based scenarios on the improvement of graduating nursing students to speak up about medication errors: a quasi-experimental study. *Nurse Education Today* 87: 104359.

Last, J.M. (ed.) (1988). *A Dictionary of Epidemiology*. New York: Oxford University Press.

Long, H.A., French, D.P., and Brooks, J.M. (2020). Optimising the value of the critical appraisal skills programme (CASP) tool for quality appraisal in qualitative evidence synthesis. *Research Methods in Medicine & Health Sciences* 1 (1): 31–42.

Morrison, K. (2023). Dissecting the literature: the importance of critical appraisal. London: Royal College of Surgeons. https://www.rcseng.ac.uk/library-and-publications/library/blog/dissecting-the-literature-the-importance-of-critical-appraisal (accessed 4 December 2023).

Nursing and Midwifery Council (2018). Standards for nursing associates. https://www.nmc.org.uk/standards/standards-for-nursing-associates (accessed 4 December 2023).

Raby, P. and Jayne McNaughton, R. (2021). A simplified approach to critically appraising research evidence. *Nurse Researcher* 29 (1): 32–41. https://doi.org/10.7748/nr.2021.e1760.

Rebar, C.R. and Macnee, C.L. (2010). *Understanding Nursing Research: Using Research in Evidence-based Practice*, 3e. Philadelphia: Lippincott Williams & Wilkins.

Sharples, J.M., Oxman, A.D., Mahtani, J.R. et al. (2017). Critical thinking in healthcare and education. *BMJ* 357: j2234.

Tod, D., Booth, A., and Smith, B. (2022). Critical appraisal. *International Review of Sport and Exercise Psychology* 15 (1): 52–72. https://doi.org/10.1080/17509 84X.2021.1952471.

Whiffin, C.J. and Hasselder, A. (2013). Making the link between critical appraisal, thinking and analysis. *British Journal of Nursing* 22 (14): 831–835.

CHAPTER 7

Appraising Quantitative Research

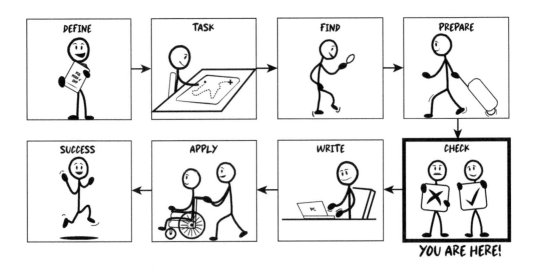

FIVE THINGS TO LEARN FROM THIS CHAPTER

1. The shared characteristics of quantitative research include objectivity, generalisability, fixed design, and numerical data.
2. Quantitative studies aim to test, measure, assess, discover, and explain.

Critical Appraisal Skills for Healthcare Students: A Practical Guide to Writing Evidence-based Practice Assignments, First Edition. Charlotte J. Whiffin, Donna Barnes, and Lorraine Henshaw.
© 2024 John Wiley & Sons Ltd. Published 2024 by John Wiley & Sons Ltd.

3. Analysis in quantitative research can either describe the data or infer the relationships between certain characteristics, events, or outcomes.
4. The quality markers in quantitative research are objectivity, validity, reliability, and generalisability.
5. The overarching concern in a quantitative study is bias.

FIVE MINUTES WITH ARJAN, ASSISTANT PRACTITIONER STUDENT

Why did you choose a quantitative study for your assignment?
I chose my quantitative study because it was relevant to my clinical role and interest, and my personal interest. I also feel like I have a numerical mindset and so the contents of the paper suited me better – I could understand the idea that data could show improvement or compare different rates (for example, wound healing) or interventions. Analysing the numbers and statistics for me made it more understandable.

What did you find hardest about appraising your paper?
I found it difficult to ensure I wasn't putting my own opinion forward although there were a lot of sources available and if you put the time in to read them, they can be used to validate and support your own appraisal points. Having some clinical experience is of course helpful in academic work but it can get in the way of appraising a research paper in which you, much like the research itself, should limit bias as much as possible.
   The data itself was also initially difficult to understand and it required learning about data types and methods to understand the outcome properly.

What strategies helped you to complete your appraisal?
Choosing a paper that relates to your work and personal interest stimulates you to keep working on the paper and learning about the topic for your own professional development.

Referring to a range of sources helped me to understand and discuss the quality issues – I found that there was actually a lot of resources available to be able to appraise quantitative research.

Although the general terminology was difficult to understand, the more classes I attended and the more reading I did around quantitative research, the more I began to understand. This then gave me the ability to appraise appropriately.

What advice do you have for anyone appraising quantitative research?

Choose a study that you are interested in, whether clinically or personally, as it will make the assignment more enjoyable and rewarding. It will also mean that you have enough knowledge to fully understand what is being measured.

However, do not get caught up with the data too much, as reading the paper will explain the results, even if you do not fully understand the data initially.

I would also advise others to read around both quantitative and qualitative to fully understand the difference between them, better understand the terminology, and be clear in your work.

Utilising the reading list and other resources provided through the module was very helpful also. Use them to do some work each week because if you can keep on top of things then when it comes to writing the essay at the end, you will already have a lot done and can then just expand on it.

7.1 INTRODUCTION

So far in this text, you have learned that for research evidence to be used effectively, it must be appraised for its quality and how well it can be applied to a particular population or context. You have also discovered that there are different approaches to research, called methodologies, that collect and analyse data in different ways, to answer different types of questions. Mann (2003) said, 'While an appropriate choice of study design is vital, it is not sufficient. The hallmark of good research is the rigour with which it is conducted.' Therefore, these next two chapters will give you an understanding and ability to appraise research methods so that you can demonstrate your skills of critical analysis within a written assignment. We will show you how in Chapter 9.

In this chapter we will first explore the common principles of good-quality quantitative research, incorporating some key principles of its appraisal, before ending with Key Facts about several specific quantitative designs to help you appraise specific types of quantitative research. This is quite a long chapter that introduces a lot of new topics. It is fair to say that many students struggle with quantitative critique and some even make an active decision to avoid it altogether. However, avoiding something because it appears to be difficult is not a good reason not to try it! We have tried to focus on the essentials in this chapter to introduce you to the key points. For a more advanced understanding you can supplement this text with the additional resources we signpost you to.

If you only need to appraise one study or one type of research design, you may want to read the main part of this chapter and then go directly to the Key Facts sheet for the type of research you have. We have assumed that some people will do this, so we have repeated key points in the different fact sheets where necessary so none of these are missed.

 Checkpoint Activity

Aim: To reflect on the limitation of information in the public domain

Instructions: Imagine for a moment you are reading the news on social media. You see the following headlines:

- Most teenagers think Sherlock Holmes was real.
- Married women drink more.
- 82% of people do not trust the results of surveys.

What would you want to know about the evidence behind these claims? For example, would it make a difference how many people were asked or where they were from?

7.2   CHARACTERISTICS OF QUANTITATIVE RESEARCH

Quantitative research deals with positive facts and observable phenomena. It subscribes to the 'scientific method', its primary goal being description, prediction, and explanation through the use of measurable evidence. It involves the collection and description of numerical data that can be interpreted through statistical testing to check whether the results found are due to chance or it is likely that the observed effect is actually real (Table 7.1).

7.2.1   Typical Quantitative Aims

Quantitative studies are usually designed to quantify and summarise the phenomena of interest or to explore the relationships that exist between variables. Therefore, a typical aim may be:

- To describe the characteristics of the phenomena of interest.
- To test whether a hypothesis is true.
- To find out if a new intervention or treatment works and to what extent.

TABLE 7.1   Shared characteristics of quantitative research.

	Objectivity	Quantitative studies provide knowledge that is as objective as possible. They try to prove or disprove ideas and concepts, outcomes, and effects to add to our knowledge and understanding. They do this through measuring factual information, based on observation or experiment, in an objective and systematic way. They then use statistical tests and modelling to try to show that their results are not simply down to a chance finding but are more likely to be true.
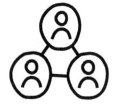	Generalisability	The point of quantitative research is that the result of the study should be generalisable to the wider population and not just the people in the study. This is ensured through a careful rigorous study design and particular consideration of the sample of participants. The sampling methods used gathers information (data) from a number of participants. The data are then analysed and the results extrapolated, making the assumption that the findings will continue in other situations and contexts.
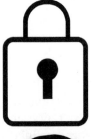	Fixed	In a quantitative study once the design is finalised it should not be adapted in any way, except for ethical and safety reasons. The rigidity and systematic nature of quantitative research ensure that the design is not compromised. This is important so that it does not introduce any external factors that could affect the study results.
	Numerical data	Statistics are common to all quantitative designs and are key to the ability of the study to provide robust, generalisable findings (this is the key purpose of quantitative research).

- To determine if a relationship exists between variables.
- To discover how often and when something occurs.

These aims are often captured by research questions commonly written as:

- Does x cause y?
- How many/much/often?
- What is the relationship between. . .?
- What is the difference between. . .?
- What are the risk factors associated with. . .?

To meet these aims of testing, comparing, and describing, quantitative research needs appropriate methods.

 Assignment Tip

You will demonstrate your understanding of quantitative research better if you *apply* your explanation of its typical characteristics and aims to the research you are appraising. If you simply describe them, it makes it harder for you to provide any analysis.

Compare these two examples, the first being descriptive, the second applied:

- Quantitative research uses numerical data and typically aims to test if a new treatment works (Whiffin et al. 2024).
- Quantitative research uses numerical data and typically aims to test if a new treatment works (Whiffin et al. 2024). This was an appropriate methodology for Smith et al.'s (2020) study*, as they collected numerical data on depression symptom severity scores, with the aim of measuring if a new drug decreased symptom severity in males aged 20–40.

* Smith et al. (2020) is a hypothetical study.

7.2.2   Typical Quantitative Data Types and Typical Data Collection Methods

The data collected in quantitative research can be measured, counted, or given a numerical value, so that it always has a numerical form (even data that may look qualitative, like free-text responses in a questionnaire, are usually quantified for analysis). However, there are different types of numerical data. Understanding the different types is important because different types of data require different analytical methods.

TABLE 7.2 Types of data in quantitative studies.

Data type	Examples	
Nominal	Only two possible answers (dichotomous) or multiple-choice questions (MCQ). **Examples**: Yes/no Marital status Gender Hair colour	Both nominal and ordinal data are called 'discrete data' or categorical data, i.e. separate, distinct values or categories
Ordinal	Rank (ordering) or scale (Likert) **Examples:** On a scale of 1–5 how hard is critical appraisal? Rank five biscuit types from least to most preferred.	
Interval	Measurement scales without a true zero[a] **Examples:** Temperature IQ Shoe size	Both are called continuous data, i.e. a continuous range of values
Ratio	Measurement scale with a true zero[a] **Examples:** Age Income Height	

[a] A true zero means a value where zero equals nothing. Temperature measured in Celsius and Fahrenheit is a good example of interval data because 0° does not mean there is no temperature. However, compare this to height where 0 cm does equal no height. Where there is a true zero, as in ratio data, accurate ratios can be calculated such as 'twice the height of. . . .' or 'four times as likely to. . .'.

The different types of data can be seen in Table 7.2. These can be remembered using the mnemonic NOIR, which stands for Nominal, Ordinal, Interval, and Ratio.

These data can be collected in numerous ways, such as those described in Table 7.3.

7.2.3 Typical Quantitative Samples

In quantitative research the main goal of sampling (recruitment of participants) is to attain a sample that is representative of the population being studied. This is so that researchers can study a smaller group and produce accurate generalisations, which they can then infer onto the larger population (known as the target population) under study. The recruitment of a representative sample that mirrors the characteristics of the target population is vital to allow these generalisations to be made.

TABLE 7.3 Common quantitative data-collection methods.

Quantitative data-collection method	What are these?	Why use these?
Controlled observations	Systematic and structured method of collecting data under conditions controlled by the researchers. For example, an experiment where a change is instigated by the researchers (like providing a new intervention) and a careful (measurable) observation is made of what happens next.	Measurements are usually more accurate and consistent if made directly by the researchers. However, sometimes the measures used do not reflect real life.
Outcome measures	A measure of a specific characteristic, event, or end point such as death (mortality); the presence or absence of symptoms or diseases (morbidity); laboratory findings from tests like urinalysis; or examinations like peak flows and muscle strength.	These measures are already known to be accurate and consistent, making them a popular choice.
Patient-reported outcome measures (PROMs)	A measure that relies on information provided directly by the patient. Examples include attitudes and behaviours; likes and dislikes; knowledge; emotion and mood; health and quality of life.	Sometimes clinical outcome measures are too narrow to be meaningful, e.g. measuring the presence of cortisol in the blood as the only indicator of stress. Such a study would benefit from a PROM, which will ask a participant about their experience of feeling stress rather than relying on a blood biomarker.
Questionnaires	Sets of closed and/or open questions to gather information about a range of subjects. Can be completed online, over the phone, in person, or as a hard copy sent in the post. The participant can self-fill the questionnaire or it can be completed by the researcher for the participant.	A good way to quickly generate a lot of data. There are lots of questionnaires already made that can be reused or researchers can make their own for the study. Researchers need to consider the content and structure of the questions. They should also test a questionnaire out before sending it to the main study sample.
Document review	Data collected from documents that already exist, e.g. reports, meeting minutes, patient records, public records, and audit data. Increasingly popular since the growth of digital technology in health.	An efficient and manageable way to collect data from past events. Some of the documents will be already in the public domain and are easily accessible to researchers; others such as patient records are more difficult to access and will require consent.

Research Essentials

Study sample: people/participants in the study.

Target population: people not in the study who the study sample are supposed to represent.

Generalisation: making a claim as to whether the results found in the study sample are likely to be true for the target population.

There are some important considerations when recruiting a sample:

- **Size:** When the sample size is too small it is less likely to reflect the target population and this in turn reduces its generalisability. Big samples are preferred because they are more likely to reflect the target population and thus increase the study's generalisability. But how big is big enough? To find out, researchers can conduct a **power calculation**.
- **Range:** The sample needs to reflect the range of characteristics in the target population. All variables that are considered important should be represented, so check who took part.
- **Over/under-representation:** The sample should be well balanced in terms of certain characteristics. There should not be over- or under-representation of one or more types of participants. For example clinical trials are often conducted on healthy men. Also consider groups who are missed from research. The NIHR (2024) calls these under served groups and includes factors such as age, sex, ethnicity and education, as well as social and economic factors.

 Research Essentials

Power calculations: A power calculation will estimate how many participants are needed. These are typically used where researchers are looking for significant differences, relationships, or associations between variables. When studies do not have a large enough sample they are described as being 'underpowered'.

Quantitative researchers often use a method of sampling called 'probability sampling', but they can also use 'non-probability' methods for some types of quantitative research.

In probability sampling the quantitative researcher first considers the 'target population' or the population of interest. This could be people with type 2 diabetes, or adults who are medically obese. Each of the individuals in the target population then has an equal chance of being selected for the study. Using probability sampling will mean that that study sample is more likely to represent the main characteristics of the target population. Therefore, findings that are true for the sample are more likely to be true for the target population.

There are several different ways to undertake probability sampling. These are explained in Table 7.4.

In contrast, non-probability sampling uses non-random techniques to select a sample. These methods are more common in qualitative studies, but quantitative researchers may also use them. Without probability sampling techniques, results cannot be generalised. Despite this, these methods can still prove useful in quantitative research, such as in the following circumstances:

- When it is difficult to be sure who is in the target population.
- When the results are only relevant to a particular group or organisation.

TABLE 7.4   Types of probability sampling.

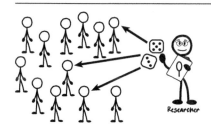

Random sampling

Random sampling is used to select participants from a list of the target population. This ensure that each person has an equal chance of being selected for the study. Random sampling can be decided from something as simple as a coin toss or pulling names from a hat, to more sophisticated randomisation using random number generators to identify participants for recruitment.
Considerations: It is difficult to ensure that every person is on the target population list in the first place. May still lead to under- or over-representation of certain groups.

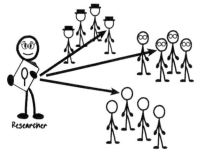

Stratified sampling

Stratified sampling helps to reduce the likelihood of over/under-representation of certain groups.
The target population is organised into subgroups (called 'strata') and people are selected randomly from each of these, meaning equal recruitment from each subgroup. The researcher chooses the subgroups based on their importance or relevance to the research question.
Considerations: Useful to ensure the sample is representative of important characteristics in the target population.
May be 'weighted' so that more people from certain subgroups are recruited, for example including more people from a particular age range where the research findings may be more pertinent.

(Continued)

TABLE 7.4   (Continued)

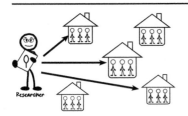

Cluster sampling

In cluster sampling the target population is 'clustered' into groups.

Usually, these clusters already exist naturally.

For example, if we wanted to examine healthcare students' use of critical appraisal tools, we could randomly select universities with healthcare students and each university would be a cluster.

Considerations: Useful for larger populations where there are already predefined groups, where there are significant barriers to the same site providing two different interventions, or when there are concerns that there may be contamination between the two groups.

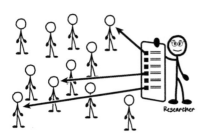

Systematic sampling

In this method the target population is listed and organised in some way, for example age of diagnosis or days in hospital.

People are then selected from the list at pre-set intervals, e.g. every tenth person, until the required number for the sample is met.

Considerations: Simple and efficient to implement Spreads the sample throughout the target population more evenly.

- When random sampling is not feasible or practical.
- Where the research is exploratory.
- Where the study is a pilot study.

Non-probability sampling includes, purposive, convenience, and snowball sampling. Check out Chapter 8 for further information on these techniques.

7.2.4   Typical Quantitative Data Analysis Methods

We will now describe some of the main data analysis techniques in quantitative research. Before this, though, it is worth highlighting that the statistical analysis reported in the study is just one part of a quantitative study. You can make a reasonably informed judgement about the quality of quantitative studies by looking at their overall design, which includes recruitment, sampling, data-collection method, and analysis. But do not be tempted to skip past the analysis or be put off by the statistics reported in your study. You do need to check if the results support the discussion section (i.e. whether they back up what is being said) and the

---

Box 7.1   Student-Recommended Statistics Texts

Swinscow, T.D.V., and Campbell, M.J. (2002). *Statistics at Square One*. London: BMJ.

Campbell, M.J., and Jacques, R.M. (2023). *Statistics at Square Two*. Chichester: Wiley.

Hoare, Z., and Hoe, J. (2013). Understanding quantitative research: part 2. *Nursing Standard* 27 (18): 48–55.

Maltby, J., Day, L., and Williams, G. (2007). *Introduction to Statistics for Nurses*. London: Routledge.

Rumsey, D.J. (2015). *U Can: Statistics for Dummies*. Chichester: Wiley.

Salkind, N.J. (2010). *Statistics for People Who (Think They) Hate Statistics*. London: Sage.

Scott, I., and Mazhindu, D. (2014). *Statistics for Healthcare Professionals: An Introduction*. London: Sage.

---

conclusions drawn from the results. If you want to know more about statistics, we recommend the texts in Box 7.1.

There are two main types of quantitative analysis: descriptive and inferential.

7.2.4.1 Descriptive Analysis

Descriptive analysis is used to describe and summarise numerical data that provide more a useful, concise overview. Examples include averages (called measures of central tendency), frequencies (number of times), proportions (percentages), and spread (ranges) (Table 7.5).

 Aim: To understand different types of averages and how they are calculated

Instructions: Complete the following calculations.

If you have eight participants in a study and you measure their weight, you will get a list of weights in kg:

$$65, 67, 72, 78, 78, 80, 89, 95$$

Calculating the mean (the total value divided by the number of values):

$$65 + 67 + 72 + 78 + 78 + 80 + 89 + 95 = 624 / 8$$
$$\textbf{Mcan} = \textbf{78}$$

Calculating the mode (the most common value):

$$65 + 67 + 72 + \textbf{78} + \textbf{78} + 80 + 89 + 95$$
$$\textbf{Mode} = \textbf{78}$$

Calculating the median. The median is the middle value (in this case there is no explicit middle value, so this is calculated by adding the values together and dividing by two):

1	2	3	4	5	6	7	8
65	67	72	**78**	**78**	80	89	95

Median = 78

In the example you can see that the mean, mode and median are all the same. This is useful because it tells us the data are normally distributed. See Research Essentials for more information about normal distribution.

TABLE 7.5   Descriptive statistics.

Measures of central tendency	Ways of describing the centre values of the data set
	Mean: The sum of all the values in a data set added together and then divided by the number of values
	Median: The value in the middle of the data set if values are set out in order
	Mode: The most commonly occurring value
Frequencies	The number of observations that occur in the sample These may be illustrated on line and bar charts or graphs
Proportions	A part or share of the whole data set, e.g. a percentages These may be displayed as pie charts
Spread	**Range**: Provides the actual range for a value in a data set, for example the average age may be 22 but the youngest person may be 12 and the oldest 86, so the range is 12–86 **Inter-quartile range**: If we imagine the whole of a data set is ordered (low to high) and then split into quarters (chunks of 25%), then the middle 50% is the inter-quartile range It is helpful as it tells you the spread of the middle half of your distribution and it is not so affected by outliers (very low or high values) **Standard deviation (SD)**: This tells us about the average variability around the mean and is found by calculating the distance from the mean for each value in a data set It gives you an idea of the spread of the values in a data set If the SD is high, there is more overall spread from the mean value, and this can be helpful to enable you to see how diverse the scores or values from the participants are If the SD is small this this would tell you that the sample range is small and less diverse

7.2.4.2 Inferential Analysis

In contrast, inferential statistics are used to 'infer' relationships between variables in the data. Inferential statistics are used when researchers want to test hypotheses or make predictions, for example about the relationship between weight and heart disease, or loneliness and depression. Inferential statistics measure the probability of observed differences happening by chance.

 Research Essentials

Hypothesis: A statement, or prediction, about the relationship between variables. e.g. people who eat chocolate at least once a day are happier than those who do not.

Hypothesis testing: Once the initial prediction has been made, the prediction is reworded to two statements. The first states there is no relationship between variables (called a null hypothesis or H^0); the second is the 'alternative hypothesis' (or H^1) that says there is a relationship.
e.g.
H^0 = There is no difference in happiness between those who eat chocolate once every day and those that don't.
H^1 = There is a difference in happiness between those who eat chocolate once every day and those that don't.

In hypothesis testing the statistical tests actually work to disprove the null hypothesis, which allows it to be rejected. When this is the case the alternative hypothesis must be accepted as true.

There are two types of inferential statistics: parametric and non-parametric. Some examples of these are described in Table 7.6.

TABLE 7.6 Non-parametric and parametric tests.

Non-parametric tests	Typically, non-parametric tests are used on categorical data (nominal and ordinal) and where the data are not 'normally distributed'[a]	Examples	Mann–Whitney U test Chi-squared test Wilcoxon signed-rank test Kruskal–Wallis test
Parametric tests	These are powerful statistical tests and come with strict rules about their use Rule 1: Should only be used on interval and ratio data (not everyone agrees on this point!) Rule 2: Should only be used when the researchers are confident that the data are 'normally distributed'	Examples	T-test Paired T-test ANOVA (analysis of variance) ANCOVA (analysis of covariance)

[a] Normal distribution means that the data vary in a predictable way around the average value. Normally distributed data create a 'bell-shaped curve' that has the same distribution either side of the average value. If you want to understand this is in more detail, see the Research Essentials box.

Research Essentials

Normal distribution: This is an important concept in statistical analysis as the normal distribution of data sets allows researchers to decide which types of statistical tests are appropriate. They may not mention this in a study specifically, but they may describe undertaking parametric or non-parametric statistical methods. The decision to use these is based on this concept.

A normal distribution is often defined if the mean, mode, and median of the data set are the same. If data of this type were plotted on a graph, this would produce a bell-shaped curve. For example, if we think about the height of a sample and plot the height of all the individuals in that sample, we will get a graph that looks like this:

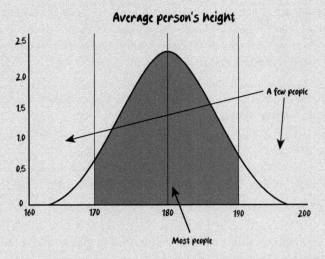

This is known as a bell-shaped curve and it signifies the normal distribution of data.

7.2.5   Typical Quantitative Findings

When reading a quantitative study, the first thing you may see is a table of participant characteristics (called demographics). This is important because it allows you to see who took part in the study and if there are any differences between them that may affect the study results.

Checkpoint Activity

Aim: To explore demographic data and look for potential concerns

Instructions: In the following table you will see some fictitious study data. Take a closer look at the data. Can you spot any potential issues?

- Are the two groups similar for all variables?
- Are the counts accurate?

		Overall (n = 400)	Intervention group (n = 200)	Control group (n = 200)
Age range (yr) (mean)	<25	0	0	0
	25–35	0	0	0
	36–46	20	9	11
	46–55	60	27	33
	56–65	120	62	58
	66–75	140	71	69
	76–85	140	72	68
	86–95	120	59	61
	95+	10	4	6
Weight (kg) (mean)		85	90	80
Sex	Male	219	111	108
	Female	179	87	92
	Not recorded	2	0	2
Smoking status	Never	215	113	102
	Previously	95	48	47
	Currently	100	48	52
	Not recorded	3	1	2
Previous coronary event	Stroke	140	46	94
	Myocardial infarction	260	155	95

Answer: Look at the data reported for smoking status. The totals of these columns add up to 413, not 400 as stated as the overall number of participants (n = 400). This reporting error would suggest further inaccuracies. Also look at the amounts in the control and intervention groups – do these match the overall for each category of smoking status?

Now look at the data for 'previous coronary event'. The intervention and control groups should be the same (or very similar). However, you can see that the intervention group has a lot more participants with myocardial infarctions but less strokes than the control group. Therefore, there are important differences between the intervention and control groups at the start of the study, which may have an impact on the results.

The table of demographic data in a study would be followed by a series of other tables that show the results of the research and a discussion section, which should discuss the interpretation of the results.

We will now focus on the results of inferential tests. Examples include P values, effect size, and confidence intervals.

P values: When reading quantitative studies, you will commonly see the results of P values. These results are generated by the inferential statistics and tell you the results of hypothesis testing in the study. Researchers must allow for the result they calculated to have occurred by chance. For example, students with brown hair may all get firsts in their degree one year. Although this is true for the sample, is it likely to be true for the target population?

Effect size: Over the years a lot of attention has been given to P values, leading to some misinterpretation of the value of certain interventions. Therefore, in addition to the P value the researchers should also give the 'effect size'. It is actually the effect size that is more important in interpreting the value of the intervention.

Confidence Intervals: These help with the interpretation of results by giving upper and lower limits of the likely size of any effect shown in the results. They are used to show statistical significance, sometimes by themselves and sometimes with P values. They tell us more than P values, though, because they provide a range of possible values.

You can explore these concepts further by checking out the next research essentials box or further reading in the statistical texts suggested in Box 8.1.

 Research Essentials

P values: These are reported as equal to (=), less than (<), or greater than (>). The threshold at which a result is considered to be statistically significant is 0.05. This means it is unlikely (5% or less chance) that the observed result happened by chance alone.

P values tell you how likely it is that there is a difference between two groups. However, they do not describe by how much.

Effect size: This is the size (or magnitude) of difference between two groups. P values will identify whether an effect exists, e.g. whether it is likely that the intervention causes the outcome, but they will not provide any information on the size of the effect. Therefore, the intervention may make some difference to the outcome, but if that difference is very small it may not be worth investing in the new intervention.

Confidence intervals: These indicate a range within which the true value in a population sits. The confidence interval (CI) is also presented with a percentage chance that the range contains this true value. This is known as the confidence level (CL) and often is given as 95%. Results must be written to show both CL and CI, for example:

The average number of hours for which children watch TV in 1 week is 34 h, 95% CI (26–42 h)

Confidence intervals are normally set at 95%. However, they can be smaller and this usually will provide you with a narrower range in which the true population value sits, i.e. for the current example this might be 50% CI (32–36 h) or a larger range with a 99% CI (23–47 h) (Pezzullo 2013).

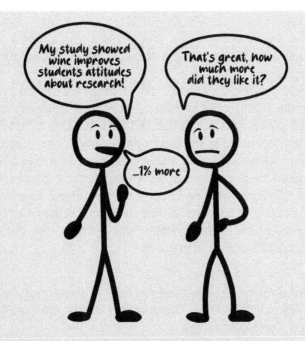

Statistical significance is the least interesting thing about the results. You should describe the results in terms of measures of magnitude – not just, does a treatment affect people, but how much does it affect them.

Gene v. Glass cited in Sullivan and Feinn (2012, p. 279)

Table 7.7 describes some additional statistical concepts and tests that you may come across when reading a quantitative study. Some of these are explored further in the Key Facts sheets. However, there are more that are beyond the scope of this text.

TABLE 7.7   More statistical tests.

Cohen's d	This is the most common way to measure effect size Cohen's d is the standardised mean difference between two groups
Odds ratio (OR)	An OR measures the relationship between an exposure to something and an outcome, for example diet and heart disease A confidence interval is used to signify the precision of the OR If the odds of the outcome are the same in both groups the OR is 1
Risk ratio/relative risk (RR)	This calculates, and then compares, the risk of disease or event in one group of people with the risk of the same disease or event in another group If the RR is 1 there is the same risk in both groups
Number needed to treat (NNT)	This is the number of people who need to be treated to prevent one event, e.g. we need to treat 10 people to prevent 1 person becoming unwell

7.2.6   Examples

You can now see how the characteristics of quantitative research play out in the following two examples.

In the first example from Jones et al. (2016), the researchers wanted to find out if lung ultrasonography (LUS) could be used as a substitute for chest radiography (CXR) in the diagnosis of pneumonia in children. If LUS was found to be feasible and effective, it could be recommended as the imaging modality of choice given its portability and reduced healthcare costs. The researchers chose an experimental design with participants randomised to receive either LUS (intervention group) or CXR (control group). The study findings showed there were no missed cases of pneumonia in the intervention group, or differences in adverse events. If the new intervention is the same in terms of effectiveness but cheaper and easier to use, this makes a strong argument for its implementation in practice.

Feasibility and Safety of Substituting Lung Ultrasonography for Chest Radiography When Diagnosing Pneumonia in Children: A Randomized Controlled Trial

Abstract

Background

Chest radiography (CXR) is the test of choice for diagnosing pneumonia. Lung ultrasonography (LUS) has been shown to be accurate for diagnosing pneumonia in children and may be an alternative to CXR. Our objective was to determine the feasibility and safety of substituting LUS for CXR when evaluating children suspected of having pneumonia.

Methods

We conducted a randomized control trial comparing LUS with CXR in 191 children from birth to 21 years of age suspected of having pneumonia in an ED. Patients in the investigational arm underwent LUS. If there was clinical uncertainty after ultrasonography, physicians had the option to perform CXR. Patients in the control arm underwent sequential imaging with CXR followed by LUS. The primary outcome was the rate of CXR reduction; secondary outcomes were missed pneumonia, subsequent unscheduled health-care visits, and adverse events between the investigational and control arms.

Results

There was a 38.8% reduction (95% CI, 30.0%–48.9%) in CXR among investigational subjects compared with no reduction (95% CI, 0.0%–3.6%) in the control group. Novice and experienced physician-sonologists achieved 30.0% and 60.6% reduction in CXR use, respectively. There were no cases of missed pneumonia among all study participants (investigational arm, 0.0%: 95% CI, 0.0%–2.9%; control arm,

0.0%: 95% CI, 0.0%–3.0%), or differences in adverse events, or subsequent unscheduled health-care visits between arms.

Conclusions
It may be feasible and safe to substitute LUS for CXR when evaluating children suspected of having pneumonia with no missed cases of pneumonia or increase in rates of adverse events.

Source: Jones et al. (2016)/with permission of Elsevier.

In the second example by Coto et al. (2020), the researchers wanted to quantify the impact of COVID-19 on Allied Health Professionals (AHPs) in the USA. The outcomes of interest were specified as the work environment, access to personal protective equipment (PPE), and levels of stress. Coto et al. (2020) designed their own questionnaire to collect this data as they claim no relevant questionnaire existed that they could use. Over 900 people completed the online survey and inferential statistics were used to analyse the data. The data suggest that a large proportion of AHPs felt stressed, but those with access to mental health support reported lower stress levels than those without.

The Impact of COVID-19 on Allied Health Professions

Abstract
The purpose of the current study was to examine the impact of Severe Acute Respiratory Syndrome Coronavirus 2 (SARS-CoV-2 or COVID-19) on allied health professionals work environment, access to personal protective equipment (PPE) and COVID-19 testing, and mental health. A 34-question survey was developed and distributed electronically to allied health professionals through listservs of professional organizations and social media groups. A total of 921 responses from allied health professionals in a variety of work settings were analyzed. The majority of allied health professionals had access to medical-grade PPE and agreed with their clinics decisions to stay open or closed. Private practices appeared to be the most negatively impacted with regards to employment in the form of pay reductions, furloughs, lay-offs, or the requirement of using paid time off. Importantly, 86% of all respondents, irrespective of employment status, reported feeling stressed with regards to changes in their work environment and transmission of the virus. However, levels of stress were dependent upon access to PPE and mental health resources. Specifically, those with access to mental health support reported lower stress levels than those without such access. These results highlight the need for continuous monitoring of mental health for allied health professionals in order to inform clinic and hospital policies for PPE and the development of brief interventions to mitigate adverse long-term mental health outcomes.

Source: Coto et al. (2020) / PLOS / CC BY 4.0.

Aim: To reflect on the aims and methods of quantitative research.

Checkpoint Activity

Instructions: Think for a minute about the first example. Do you understand why this study was conducted using quantitative methods? Do you think it was the right way to answer the research question? Do you understand the concepts mentioned in the abstract, such as control arm, secondary outcomes, and confidence intervals? Do you think the findings are useful?

Now think about the second example. Can you see why a quantitative approach to this research question was used? Do you think this was the right approach? What questions might you have about the questionnaire the researchers designed? What questions might you have about the study results? This study took place in the USA, do you think it is applicable to the UK?

7.3   TYPICAL QUALITY MARKERS FOR QUANTITATIVE RESEARCH

7.3.1   Objectivity, Validity, Reliability, Generalisability

Now you understand the principles of quantitative design. We will now explain the four quality markers for quantitative research. Table 7.8 will be helpful for you to return to when you need a refresher.

Assignment Tip

You will demonstrate your understanding of research quality better if you *apply* the quality markers, rather than listing them. Students often worry that they may miss something essential in an assignment and listing important concepts can feel like a way of addressing this. However, listing can only be descriptive and does not show your marker that you actually know what those concepts mean. Consider taking the most pertinent issues from your list and weaving them into separate points through your assignment.

Compare these two examples, the first a descriptive list, the second applying the criteria:

- Quantitative research has four main quality markers: objectivity, validity, reliability and generalisability (Whiffin et al. 2024).
- Good-quality quantitative research should use valid methods (Whiffin et al. 2024). Smith et al.'s (2020) study* demonstrated validity by using a well-established scale for measuring depression symptoms, which had been shown to be accurate in several previous studies.

* Smith et al. (2020) is a hypothetical study.

TABLE 7.8   Explanation of quality markers in quantitative research.

Quality marker	Think of this as. . .	Explanation
Objectivity	Impartial/free from bias	Objectivity in research is about removing the influence of any factors that could make the results less truthful through bias or contamination. Objectivity is observing (measuring) something without influencing it in any way, to get as close to the truth as possible.
Validity	Accuracy	Validity is how well any test, questionnaire, or tool we use to measure something in research accurately measures what it is trying to.
Reliability	Consistency	Reliability is how likely it is that the measurement tool (test, questionnaire, or tool) used provides the same results over and over. It is related to validity, but differs in that something can be reliable because it gives you the same results over and over, but the tool being used may not accurately measure the outcome of interest e.g. a clock which is always half an hour slow may be consistent but it is not accurate. So a test or measure can be reliable but is not necessarily valid.
Generalisability	Applicability to the target population	Generalisability is the degree to which the study participants are similar or representative to the wider group of people being researched to allow us to apply the results of the study to them (i.e. all diabetics). It is important to realise that this is not everyone in the population per se, but only the population being studied (i.e. it is restricted to people who have the same conditions, problems, etc. that are being researched). Being generalisable is a key purpose of quantitative research as it makes the research more useful. To ensure generalisability, quantitative research design considers the number and type of participants needed. The number needed is often high, which helps maintain representativeness of the wider group of people being researched through the size of the sample.

Aim: To understand quality criteria in quantitative research

Checkpoint Activity

Instructions: Don't worry if these terms seem a bit difficult to get your head round, lots of people find them tricky. Take a moment to think about what these terms mean to you. Write your own definition in the spaces provided.

Objectivity means

....

....

Validity means

....

....

Reliability means

....

....

Generalisability means

....

....

In Box 7.2 we now show you how to apply these concepts to a real study.

Box 7.2   Illustrating the Quality Criteria for Quantitative Research

A quantitative study was designed to answer the question 'How effective is a high dose of the drug Simvastatin in reducing the level of cholesterol and further coronary events?' (SEARCH Study Collaborative Group 2007).

The methods used were a clinical (experimental) trial of simvastatin at an increased dose of 80 mg, comparing it with the standard cholesterol-lowering dose of 20 mg. The outcome measures included cholesterol (low-density lipids, LDL), liver function tests (to identify possible side effects), and any coronary events (myocardial infarction and cerebrovascular accident). The participants were followed up for at least five years.

To ensure the research question was answered as accurately as possible (**validity**) the researchers needed to ensure the comparison was fair (**objectivity**) and the increased dose and standard dose were given to two similar groups of people. That is, both groups had previously had a coronary event diagnosed and also had the same balance of characteristics, such as predisposing illnesses or conditions and other factors such as age, sex, etc. The clinical trial was then designed in a way that measured the effectiveness of both doses by ensuring each dose of the drug is taken in the same way by each participant, for the same duration, increasing objectivity. The only difference was that the control group took 20 mg simvastatin, whereas the intervention group took 80 mg.

The effectiveness of each dose was tested by observing the physiological measures of LDL and a long follow-up of at least five years to record future incidence of any coronary events and other factors such as side effects. The LDL measure was checked at the same time intervals for every patient in the study (i.e. every 3 months in year 1, every 6 months in years 1–5) and was taken in the same way and using the same test (i.e. fasting cholesterol) (**reliability**); it was also a test that is proven to accurately measure LDL (**validity**). As well as the two groups of participants in the study being similar, the whole study population was comparable in nature to the wider population who had had a previous coronary event, with a balance of characteristics across all. This meant the results of the study would be more likely to apply to all people with a previous coronary event (**generalisability**), making the study more useful.

Note: This study was among a number of others that measured the effectiveness of lowering LDL concentrations and provided evidence that a lower LDL does reduce the risk of major vascular events, with intensive LDL lowering reducing this risk even further. However, the study also provided evidence that intensive lowering with the increased dose (80 mg) of simvastatin led to a significant increase in the risk of muscle pain (myopathy), a known side effect, of around 10 times (1 in 1000 patients/yr). The level of risk for the standard dose was 1 in 10000 patients/yr. The study led to the identification of a genetic variant present in many of the participants who developed myopathy. Subsequently it was recommended that other cholesterol-lowering regimens were used for intensive LDL-lowering needs.

Source: Adapted from Armitage et al. (2010).

7.3.2   The Overarching Concern in Quantitative Research: Bias

Now you have an explanation of the main quality markers, we need to look a little more closely at the term 'bias'. Bias is a key issue in quantitative research and if it is not controlled it can drastically affect the results and ultimately undermine the quality of any study.

 Assignment Tip

We find that when students talk about bias in an assignment, they tend to think of bias as just one thing. While bias can be considered a generic umbrella term to refer to anything that reduces our confidence in the accuracy of the results, there are lots of specific types of bias. So be clear what type of bias it is that you are concerned about.

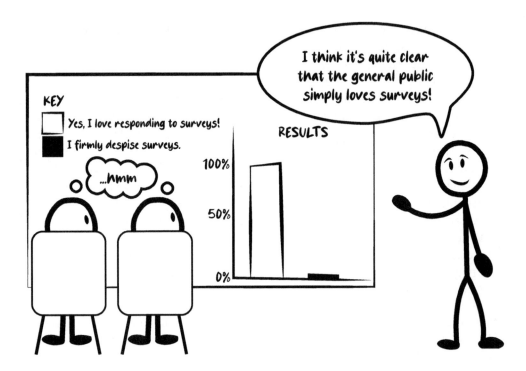

Table 7.9 describes six different types of bias. These biases affect the validity, reliability, and generalisability of a study and they are important when appraising quantitative research.

 Explore It!

If you want to look at bias in more detail, the Catalogue of Bias is a great website to explore: www.catalogofbias.org

7.4 QUANTITATIVE DESIGNS KEY FACTS SHEETS

Now you understand quality markers and, more specifically, bias in quantitative research, we are going to look at different quantitative research designs, including surveys; experimental designs – randomised controlled trials (RCTs) and quasi-experimental (non-RCTs); cohort; and case–control studies. Each Key Facts Sheet will provide a quick overview of the design, its aims, and typical research questions with some real examples. Three unique design features are then described followed by the EDECA appraisal considerations. A mini glossary is given and some key resources if you want a more advanced understanding.

TABLE 7.9   Types of bias.

	Introduced through. . .	Examples
Measurement bias	The use of measurement tools that are not able to provide an accurate assessment of the characteristic/factor being examined.	If we use a questionnaire to measure happiness that has not been established as a valid way of measuring how happy people feel. If we use a blood pressure monitor that has not been calibrated.
Selection bias	The selection of participants is not representative of the population being studied. The allocation of participants to different groups in a study, for the purpose of comparing, is not based on the same characteristics.	If the population being studied is all adult diabetics and the age range of the study participants is over 60 only. If the groups of participants differ in terms of ethnicity, e.g. group 1 (intervention group) = 80% white British, group 2 (control group) = 50% white British.
Confirmation bias	Awareness by the participants and researcher of the intervention being received by a participant. This may cause them to report the outcomes of this intervention more favourably if they believe this intervention is the best one.	If a new drug for Alzheimer's shows promising results already and you as a researcher strongly believe that this drug will be beneficial and needs to be widely available, you may be more likely to report the effect of the drug favourably, downplaying the negatives such as side effects.
Recall bias	The participants in a study being asked to recall events or symptoms, etc., where this recollection is not a true reflection of the event.	If you ask someone to recall symptoms such as frequency of headaches and they remember this incorrectly, skewing the results of the study.
Expectancy bias	Participants or researchers reporting differently because of what they think might be the desired response.	If participants in a trial of a new drug report that it is having more of an effect because they expect it will. Similarly, if researchers also report more positive responses from participants and less negative or vice versa.
Hawthorne effect	Participants acting differently because they are part of the study.	If in a study to explore the typical exercise regime in patients with osteoarthritis, the participants in the study do more exercise than usual because they are in the study and hence skew the results.

7.4.1   Surveys

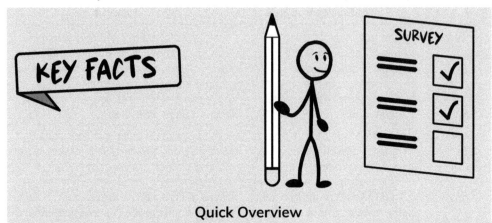

Quick Overview

Note: Survey designs can be qualitative or quantitative or mixed methods. This section is focused on quantitative surveys only.

- Survey designs include several different methods of data collection, the most common being the questionnaire. Be aware that the terms survey and questionnaires are often used interchangeably but there is a difference.
- Surveys can also be completed using observations and through interviews.
- Survey designs are very popular in healthcare and wider society. The ease with which researchers can collect data using questionnaires makes this an attractive method for those who do not need a lot of complex, in-depth information.
- Surveys can be descriptive or inferential.
- Descriptive surveys aim to describe patterns in the data set without analysis of why these patterns exist.
- Inferential surveys aim to identify relationships in the data. These are called correlational and comparative surveys (Hasson et al. 2010).

Aims: to describe or explore key characteristics of a sample with the aim of applying these findings to a wider population.
Typical research question: What are the . . . (attitudes, behaviours, health status) of the population of interest?

Real Examples

- Survey of occupational therapy students' attitudes towards sexual issues in clinical practice (Jones et al. 2005).
- A survey into student nurses' attitudes towards mental illness (Schafer et al. 2011).

- Allied health professionals' perceptions of research in the United Kingdom national health service: a survey of research capacity and culture (Comer et al. 2022).

Three Unique Design Issues

1. **Robust design and testing**

   If the survey is poor, the data will be equally poor (rubbish in, rubbish out). In questionnaire methods the researchers must convince you that the questionnaire is 'valid' and 'reliable'. Luckily there are lots of pre-validated questionnaires available that can be used to measure a number of important factors in healthcare, e.g. patient satisfaction or quality of life.

   Make a note of these four different types of validity in questionnaire designs: content, face, criterion, and construct.

   - Think of 'face validity' as 'on the face of it, but without formally checking, the questionnaire seems to ask questions that are relevant'.
   - Think of 'content validity' as 'the content of this questionnaire has been checked by experts to make sure it is relevant'.
   - Think of criterion validity as 'the questionnaire has been checked against a widely accepted "criterion" for the concept being measured'.
   - Think of construct validity as 'the questionnaire has been compared to other questionnaires that measure similar "constructs"'.

   Some questionnaires that want to measure specific outcomes like anxiety and depression will have gone through rigorous testing to establish validity (check out the Hospital Anxiety and Depression Scale; Zigmond and Snaith 1983). Other questionnaires are designed specifically for the study and will not have criterion or construct validity, but they should at least have face or content validity as these are easier to ascertain.

   Questionnaires also need to be reliable. Reliability for a questionnaire means that participants always interpret the questions in the same way. An easy way of knowing if the questionnaire is reliable is to ask participants to complete the same questionnaire twice. The consistency between scores at these two time points can be tested using a reliability coefficient like test–retest or 'Cronbach alpha' (see Mini Glossary).

2. **Response rates**

   Data-collection methods that rely on people completing and returning questionnaires are often undermined because some do not respond. The number of people who do respond divided by the number of people who were asked is called the response rate. Response rates of 75% and over are considered good (Bowling 2002). However, researchers typically report much lower response rates. The ability of a survey design to make generalisations depends on how representative the research sample is of the larger population. If the sample is not representative, any inferences made to this larger population may not be valid.

3. **Response format**

Questions can be 'open' or 'closed'. Open questions allow participants to 'freestyle' and write any comments they like. These are useful for more detailed information that the research may not be able to predict in advance. However, they do take longer for participants to complete and for the researcher to analyse. Therefore, more commonly response formats are 'closed'. Closed questions are those where there are a number of limited options to choose from, like 'yes/no' or 'strongly agree to strongly disagree', and categories including age, sex, and marital status.

Strengths

- Good for reaching a large number of people, often quickly, and relatively inexpensively.

Limitations

- If badly designed the results may not be valid or reliable.
- Can be significantly affected by a low response rate, which affects their generalisability.

EDECA Appraisal Considerations

Ethics

- Was appropriate ethical approval/favourable opinion granted for the study?
- Was completion of the survey anonymous?

Design

- Was a survey design the best way to answer the research question?

Enrol

- Who was the intended sample and are they representative of the population being studied? Hint – look at the demographic information.
- How many people were invited to complete the data-collection method and how many responded (response rate)? Hint – this will be provided as a percentage; rates of 75% and over are considered good.
- Is the final study sample still representative of the larger population? Hint – Did those who respond differ in any important way from those who did not respond to the survey?

Collect

- How did they know their data-collection methods were appropriate for the study? Hint – check if they used 'validated measures' or if they designed these themselves. If they designed them themselves, check if any of the methods were piloted prior to the main study.
- Were the questions clear and unambiguous? Hint – check to see if the questions are reported in the paper, and use your judgement to see if they seem appropriate.
- How do you know if the tool was valid? Hint – check for any reference to face, content, criterion, or construct validity.
- How do you know if the tool was reliable? Hint – check for 'test–retest' and reliability coefficients like Cronbach alpha. Remember, any coefficient above 0.7 is considered good.

Analyse

- Was the analysis of data descriptive or inferential and does this seem to be the best way of analysing the data?
- Are there any important descriptive statistics reported?
- Are there any inferences made about the relationship between variables? Hint – look for a P value of 0.05 or less. If you are unsure what P values are, go back in this chapter to refresh your memory or read a statistical textbook like *Statistics at Square One* (Campbell and Jacques 2023).

Mini Glossary

Criterion validity   Does the questionnaire measure the specific 'criterion' accurately?

Construct validity   Does the questionnaire accurately reflect the 'construct' under investigation?

Content validity   Do a panel of experts feel the content of the questionnaire is appropriate?

Cronbach alpha   A common reliability coefficient used to measure internal consistency.

Descriptive analysis   Describes the distribution of variables in the data set.

Face validity   Does the questionnaire measure what it is supposed to measure and how accurately does it do this on face value?

Inferential analysis   Infers relationships between variables in the data set.

Internal validity   The extent to which the study accurately determines if a relationship exists between variables.

Likert scales   An attitudinal response in a scale format.

Longitudinal   Following up the same sample over a period of time.

Outcome measure   A measure of a specific characteristic, event, or end point

Reliability   Is concerned with the ability of an instrument to measure consistently, time and time again.

Reliability coefficient   A measure of reliability (or internal consistency) obtained by determining the difference between two sets of measurements obtained from the same individuals. You may see this reported as Cronbach alpha. These results range from 0, meaning all the scores were totally different, to 1, meaning perfect alignment between the first and second scores. In reality there is rarely perfect alignment, so there is a threshold at which researchers are confident that the questionnaire is reliable enough. Obviously, the closer to 1 the better, but as a rule of thumb anything over 0.7 is considered good (Morera and Stokes 2016).

Response Rates   The number of people who respond to a survey divided by those who were invited.

Test–retest reliability   How consistent results are when multiple results are obtained from the same people (assuming nothing else has changed).

Key Resources

Comer, C., Collings, R., McCracken, A., Payne, C., and Moore, A. (2022). Allied health professionals' perceptions of research in the United Kingdom national health service: a survey of research capacity and culture. *BMC Health Services Research* 22: 1094. https://doi.org/10.1186/s12913-022-08465-6.

Coster, W.J. (2013). Making the best match: selecting outcome measures for clinical trials and outcome studies. *American Journal of Occupational Therapy* 67 (2): 162–170. https://doi.org/10.5014/ajot.2013.006015.

Hasson, F., McKenna, H., and Keeney, S. (2010). Surveys. In: *The Research Process in Nursing* (ed. K. Gerrish and A. Lacey). Chichester: Wiley, 255–266.

Hoare, Z., and Hoe, J. (2013). Understanding quantitative research: part 2. *Nursing Standard* 27 (18): 48–55. https://doi.org/10.7748/ns2013.01.27.18.48.c9488.

Jones, M., and Rattray, J. (2010). Questionnaire design. In: *The Research Process in Nursing* (ed. K. Gerrish and A. Lacey). Chichester: Wiley, 413–426.

Morera, O.F., and Stokes, S.M. (2016). Coefficient α as a measure of test score reliability: review of 3 popular misconceptions. *American Journal of Public Health* 106 (3): 458–461. https://doi.org/10.2105/AJPH.2015.302993.

Ponto, J. (2015). Understanding and evaluating survey research. *Journal of the Advanced Practitioner in Oncology* 6 (2): 168–171.

7.4.2   Experimental Designs

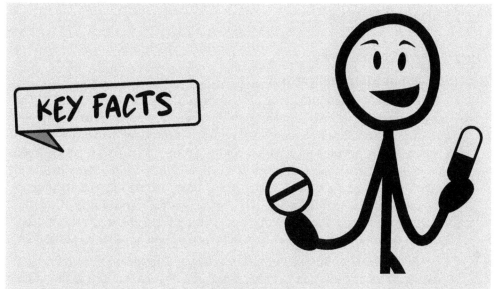

Quick Overview

- There are three main types of experimental designs: RCTs, quasi-control studies, and pre-test–post-test designs.
- Experimental designs are intervention studies where researchers actively do something (like provide a new intervention) to a group of people who would not have been exposed to this under normal circumstances. This is called **exposure**. Once participants have been exposed, data are collected to measure how they responded after being exposed. This is called the **outcome**.
- Experimental studies always move forward in time and begin prior to exposure. Exposure is then controlled by the researchers who decide when and where exposure will take place. This is called a **prospective experimental** design.
- Researchers will predict the relationship between exposure (i.e. the intervention) and the outcome by stating a **hypothesis**, e.g. 'If you stay up late (exposure) you will feel tired the next day (outcome).' The study is then designed to test the likelihood that this statement is true. This is called **causality**.

Aim: To establish the probability that exposure causes outcome.
Typical research questions: Is X more effective than Y? Does X cause Y?

Real Examples

- Postoperative packing of perianal abscess cavities (Newton et al. 2022).
- Canine assisted occupational therapy for children on the autism spectrum (Hill et al. 2020).

- Reducing distress in university students: a RCT of two online interventions (Stallman et al. 2019).

Three Unique Design Issues

1. **Randomisation and control**

   Random assignment into groups is a distinguishing feature of the RCT. The different groups in an RCT are often called 'arms'. The **study arm** is the group who are exposed to a treatment/intervention; the **control arm** is not exposed and act as a comparison (called a control group). The differences between these groups are analysed at the start of the study (called **baseline**) and then again after they have or have not been exposed to the treatment/intervention (called **follow-up**). If random assignment (**randomisation**) has worked, the groups should be the same at the start of the study, and if exposure to the intervention causes an outcome, they will be different at the end.

   Randomisation should be based on chance. This means there is an equal chance of being allocated to either the exposed (intervention) group or the unexposed (control) group (Connelly and Woolston 2016). Randomisation should be done using a random generator and not by a researcher choosing which group they place individuals in. If there are any baseline differences between groups at the start of the study, these may interfere with the experiment (called a **confounding variable**).

   However, random allocation may not be ethical, feasible, or pragmatic, for example where there is already clear evidence that exposure causes outcome, where individuals have strong beliefs or preferences, or where logistics mean it would not be possible to provide individuals with different treatments in the same environment.

   Where researchers do not use random allocation to groups this is called a 'quasi-experimental' or 'non-randomised controlled trial' (NRCT). Quasi-controlled studies are not as strong in terms of evidencing cause and effect, but sometimes there is no other way to conduct the trial. Other experimental designs of note are controlled before-and-after studies and 'pre-test–post-test' designs.

2. **Blinding**

   Blinding in experimental designs works to prevent people from knowing if they are receiving the experimental treatment/intervention. This is done to try to reduce the likelihood of a therapeutic effect due to the expectation of or belief that the treatment will be effective (called the placebo effect). An example would be acting drunk when you do not know the beer you are drinking is alcohol free!

   In some studies the participants and researchers are blinded, i.e. no one knows who is taking the experimental drug (called **double blinding**).

In other studies either the participant is blind or the researcher is blind (**single blinding**). The decision over blinding will depend on what is being tested.

3. **Statistical probability**

The whole point of an experimental design is to find out the statistical probability that exposure causes outcome. Researchers do this is a number of ways, including significance testing, effect size, and confidence intervals.

Significance testing: Earlier in this chapter you were introduced to P values. According to convention a P value that is below 5% (expressed as $P < 0.05$) is statistically significant. What this means in a clinical trial is that the difference identified between the control and study arms is unlikely to have been caused by chance (Scott and Mazhindu 2014). However, this does not automatically mean the result is important for practice.

Effect size: In contrast to simply identifying if a difference exists between the two groups, effect size compares the magnitude of the difference and if this difference is clinically relevant. Examples include relative risk or risk ratios (RR), odds ratios (OR), and numbers needed to treat (NNT); there are others. You can read more about RR in the cohort Key Facts sheet and about OR in the case–control Key Facts sheet. In this Key Facts sheet we will briefly explain why NNT is a useful figure to report in a clinical trial.

The NNT is easy to interpret and provides useful guidance for treating clinicians (McGough and Faraone 2009). It is an estimate of how many people needed to be treated to achieve the desired outcome. Where the NNT is very high there is a weak association between exposure and outcome, i.e. the treatment is less effective (e.g. NNT = 1000 means 1000 people have to be treated for one person to benefit). Where the NNT is very low there is a strong association between exposure and outcome, i.e. the treatment is more effective (e.g. NNT = 2 means only two people have to be treated for one person to benefit).

Confidence intervals: These were briefly discussed earlier in this chapter. You will commonly see confidence intervals reported in RCTs. These may be reported alongside the main result of the trial, the OR, or the RR. Confidence intervals are used because the result is the average result for the study sample. Confidence intervals are then needed to provide an estimate for the target population. The confidence interval therefore provides a range within which the real result in the population (and not just the calculated average of the sample) may lie. To evaluate the effectiveness of the intervention, the clinician must be as confident at both the upper and lower ranges of the confidence interval.

Some studies will report different types of statistics than those reported here, in which case we would recommend reading statistical textbooks like *Statistics at Square One* (Swinscow and Campbell 2002) and *Statistics at Square Two* (Campbell and Jacques 2023).

Strengths

Experimental designs with randomisation can control for confounding variables and remove or reduce many forms of bias. They are considered a very strong form of evidence and can help to examine causality.

Limitations

A lot of trust is placed in the findings of RCTs. However, randomisation does not always balance out the differences between the intervention and control groups (Deaton and Cartwright 2018). Too much control of the participants and their behaviour may prevent the study from being applicable to a real-world setting (called **external validity**).

EDECA Appraisal Considerations

Ethics

- Was appropriate ethical approval/favourable opinion granted for the study?
- Was it ethical to expose one group and not the other?
- Who was excluded from the study and was this reasonable? Hint – many experimental designs are conducted on healthy individuals and therefore these lack generalisability to people with existing medical conditions or diseases.

Design

- Were the experimental and control groups treated equally? Hint – did the control group receive as much attention as the experimental group?

Enrol

- Was there random assignment to control and experimental groups? Hint – look for random number generators.
- Are the groups the same at the start of the study in terms of important characteristics like age, sex, lifestyle?
- How many people dropped out and was this the same for the experimental and control groups?
- How many people are in the study sample and is this big enough? Hint – look for a power calculation or discussion of type I and type II errors.

Collect

- Was follow-up long enough to study the effects of the intervention?
- What instruments, tools, or markers were used to measure the outcome? Hint – look for validated outcome measures, standardised measurement tools, and clinical biomarkers.

Analyse

- Were individuals analysed in the group to which they were originally allocated? Hint – look for reference to the 'intention to treat' principle.
- How likely is it that exposure causes outcome? Hint – look for measures of effect size like numbers need to treat/harm (NNT/NNH) or statistical significance and confidence intervals.

Mini Glossary

Arm   Different groups in an experimental design (study arm gets the intervention, control arm does not)

Baseline   Analysis of the initial circumstances/current situation at the start of the study.

Causality   The concept that one thing causes another.

Blinding   Withholding knowledge of treatment allocation from participants and/or researchers.

Confidence intervals   The range within which the true value may lie.

Confounding   When an association is identified between the exposure and the outcome but in fact this is caused by something else.

Confounding factor   A variable that could provide an alternative explanation for the results, e.g. sex, additional morbidity. Confounding factors can be reduced through randomisation and adequate sample size.

Control group   The group that is not exposed to the treatment/intervention.

Effect size   The magnitude or strength of the relationship between variables.

Exposure   Any factor associated with the outcome of interest

Follow-up   Data collection after the participants have received the treatment/intervention.

Hypothesis   A statement of prediction about the relationship between variables.

Incidence rate   The rate at which the outcome occurs over a defined period.

Lost to follow-up   Participants who were initially enrolled but are no longer available for data collection.

Odds ratio   A measure of association between an exposure and an outcome

Outcome   An event or end point.

Outcome measures   The tool or variable used to measure the impact of the intervention.

Number needed to treat   The number of people who need to be treated to observe the desired outcome.

Placebo   A treatment or intervention that has no therapeutic effect. It is often disguised to appear the same as the active intervention being tested.

Placebo effect   A change in outcome due to the perception of efficacy.

Power calculation　Used to estimate how many participants are needed. Typically used where researchers are looking for significant differences, relationships, or associations between variables. When studies do not have a large enough sample they are described as being 'underpowered'.

Prospective　Methods that move forward in time

Randomisation　Allocation of individuals to experimental (study) or control group (arm) by chance alone.

Relative risk/risk ratio　The probability of an outcome in the exposed group versus the unexposed group (these terms are used interchangeably and are both abbreviated to RR).

Statistical probability　The likelihood of the difference between two groups occurring by chance.

Type I error　False positive i.e. when the researcher concludes there is a relationship between variables when in reality there isn't.

Type II error　False negative i.e. when the researcher concludes there is not a relationship between variables when in reality there is.

Key Resources

Akobeng, A.K. (2005). Understanding randomised controlled trials. *Archives of Disease in Childhood* 90 (8): 840–844.

Connelly, L.M. (2016). Understanding research. Randomised controlled trials. *MEDSURG Nursing* 25 (4): 281–282.

McGough, J.J., and Faraone, S.V. (2009). Estimating the size of treatment effects: moving beyond p values. *Psychiatry (Edgmont)* 6 (10): 21–29.

Melnyk, B.M. (2005). Evidence-based practice. Rapid critical appraisal of randomised controlled trials (RCTs): an essential skill for evidence-based practice (EBP). *Pediatric Nursing* 31 (1): 50–52.

7.4.3　Cohort Studies

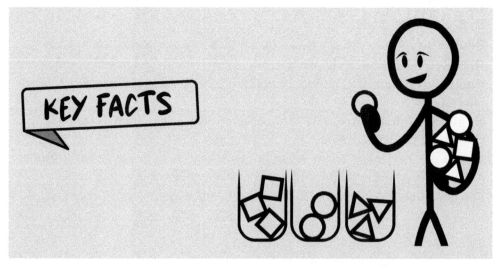

Quick Overview

- Cohort studies are observational, non-experimental studies of groups. They are usually undertaken to identify factors that might lead to a specific outcome, such as a specific disease.

- Those in the group being studied do not have the 'specific outcome' at the start of the research, but they may go on to develop it during the study (e.g. diabetes). The researchers gather data on numerous factors to try to identify frequencies or patterns in the data over time that can help to identify factors that can lead to the outcome being studied.

- Cohort studies are therefore 'longitudinal' in nature, i.e. where the same data are collected from the same people over an extended period (Barrett and Noble 2019). Most commonly cohort studies look forwards in time (prospective) or they can look back in time (retrospective), but they are always looking at the associations between exposure and outcome.

- As an observational study, a cohort study can identify relationships between variables but cannot definitively prove causation. However, it can provide very strong evidence if it is large enough.

Aim: To investigate the association between exposure to the risk factor (e.g. smoking) and the occurrence of the outcome (e.g. cancer, heart disease, diabetes).
Typical research question: What are the risk factors associated with x?

Real Examples

- Mortality associated with oral contraceptive use (Beral et al. 1999).
- Lipoprotein(a)-cholesterol and coronary heart disease (Seman et al. 1999).
- Risk factors for breast cancer according to family history of breast cancer (Colditz et al. 1996).
- Smoking and dementia in male British doctors (Doll et al. 2000).

Three Unique Design Features

1. **Large and lengthy**

   Cohort studies can be very large and include all the people born in a certain year/place/decade, etc., or sometimes they can be smaller, e.g. all the students of healthcare degree courses who completed in 2023 from a specific university. Cohort studies can collect data from thousands of people over several years. For example, a cohort study of 537 303 children recruited over seven years in Denmark found no statistical difference in the rates of autism in a groups of children who had the measles, mumps, and rubella vaccine versus children who did not (Madsen et al. 2002). However, because of the length of time involved, cohort studies can suffer from people dropping out of the study over time.

2. **Exposure assessed prior to outcome**

An important feature of a cohort study is to determine who in the cohort has been exposed to a risk factor of interest or has a characteristic of interest before the outcome occurs, for example determining if physical and mental health problems are associated with drop-out and retention among nursing students (Bakker et al. 2018). In this study three cohorts of students were followed up over 2.5 years. Initial measurements of physical and mental health were conducted at the start of the study (called 'baseline data') and then data were collected in subsequent years about drop-out from nurse education and from the nursing profession after graduation. This would be different to a study where the outcome was already known and the researchers looked back at potential risk factors that may have caused this (see case–control study Key Facts Sheet).

3. **Calculation of incidence**

In a cohort study it is unknown at the start who, and how many, will eventually have the outcome of interest. Following up the cohort over time enables the researchers to estimate the incidence of the outcome (Setia 2016). These incidence rates play a crucial role in healthcare to quantify the burden of disease, monitor disease trends, and identify risk factors. Incident rates are often presented as 'cases per 100 000 of the population'. Cohort studies may also calculate relative risk or risk ratios (RR) that compare the risk of developing the outcome between exposed and unexposed individuals in the cohort.

The risk of developing the outcome in the exposed versus unexposed groups can be expressed as a fraction. When fractions are calculated the results are *close to, greater than, or less than 1.*

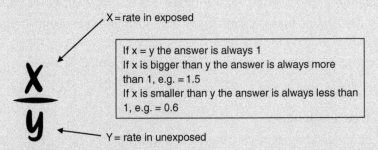

Where the RR is greater than 1 there is an increased risk of the outcome in the exposed group. Where the RR is less than 1 there is a decreased risk of the outcome in the exposed group. If the RR is 1, the risk is the same.

Therefore, the higher the RR, the greater the risk of developing the outcome in the exposed group. For example, if the RR is 10, the exposed group is 10 times more likely to develop the outcome than the unexposed group. The RR is usually presented with an accompanying confidence interval of 95% (see explanation earlier in this chapter). If the confidence interval includes 1 the study must conclude that there is no statistical difference between the groups.

Risk ratios are most commonly reported in Cohort studies. However, you may find other results cited. In that case we would recommend reading statistical textbooks like *Statistics at Square One* (Swinscow and Campbell 2002) and *Statistics at Square Two* (Campbell and Jacques 2023).

Strengths

The ability to ascertain the incidence and natural history of the outcomes of interest.

Limitations

Cohort studies are less useful to study rare events or those that take time to develop. Attrition from cohort studies is common. Where there is more or less attrition from either the exposed or unexposed group, this can cause 'attrition bias'.

EDECA Appraisal Considerations

Ethics

- Was appropriate ethical approval/favourable opinion granted for this study?
- Did people consent to be in the cohort study? Hint – some cohort studies are conducted without consent as information can be retrieved from existing sources. This may or may not be appropriate.
- Does everyone in the proposed cohort have an equal chance of being involved?

Design

- Were the 'exposure' and 'outcome' clearly defined and measurable?
- Is the measurement of exposure and outcome as objective as possible?

Enrol

- Who is the 'cohort' and how much selection bias was there? Hint – were only people at risk of the outcome included?
- Are both groups similar in all important aspects with the exception of exposure?

Collect

- Was determination of outcome made by someone who did not know if the groups were exposed or unexposed?
- Do you think the follow-up period was long enough for the outcome to be identified?
- Was any attempt made to minimise attrition?
- Was attrition similar in both exposure and unexposed groups?

Analyse

- Do the researchers identify any confounding variables? Hint – look for differences between the exposed and unexposed groups that may interfere with the results.
- Did they control for these confounding variables in the analysis? Hint – if there were confounders, look for a statement like 'we controlled for age and sex', which means that they think age and sex could be confounding variables and have accounted for this in the analysis (you do not need to know how they have done this!)

Mini Glossary

Baseline   Analysis of the initial circumstances/current situation.

Cohort   A group of participants who share a common characteristic.

Confounding   When an association is identified between the exposure and the outcome but in fact this is caused by something else.

Exposure   Any factor associated with the outcome of interest, e.g. smoking and cancer.

Incidence rate   The rate at which the outcome occurs over a defined period.

Longitudinal   Following up the same sample over a period of time.

Lost to follow-up   Participants who were initially enrolled but are no longer available for data collection.

Observational study   Documents the presence of exposure and outcomes as they occur.

Outcome   An event or end point

Prospective   Methods that move forward in time

Relative risk/risk ratio   The probability of an outcome in the exposed group versus the unexposed group (these terms are used interchangeably and are both abbreviated to RR).

Retrospective   Methods look back instead of forward.

Risk factor   Something that increases the chance of developing the outcome

Key Resources

Barrett, D., and Noble, H. (2019). What are cohort studies? *Evidence-Based Nursing* 22 (4): 95–96.

Browner, W.S., Newman, T.B., Cummings, S.R., and Grady, D.G. (2022). *Designing Clinical Research*. Philadelphia: Lippincott Williams & Wilkins.

Coggon, D., Rose, G., and Barker, D.J.P. (2003). *Epidemiology for the Uninitiated*. London: BMJ.

Grimes, D.A., and Schulz, K.F. (2002). Cohort studies: marching towards outcomes. *Lancet* 359 (9303): 341–345.

Setia, M.S. (2016). Methodology series module 1: cohort studies. *Indian Journal of Dermatology* 61 (1): 21–5. https://doi.org/10.4103/0019-5154.174011.

7.4.4   Case–Control Studies

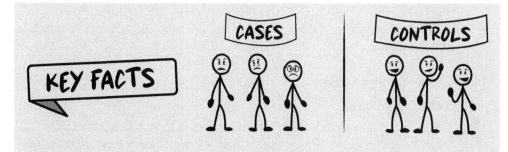

Quick Overview

- A type of observational study to examine how factors may be associated with particular outcomes of interest such as diseases/conditions (Tenny et al. 2017). Case–control studies are, by definition, always looking back to investigate exposure (i.e. retrospective) (Tenny et al. 2017).

- Useful where the incidence rate of the disease/condition of interest (called the 'outcome') is low and therefore another observational design like a cohort study may take a very long time to recruit enough people to be confident of the findings. Case–control studies are also used where an experimental design would be unethical or unfeasible.

- Case–control studies enrol people who have already developed the outcome and compare them to a group of similar people who do not have the same outcome.

- Researchers will try to identify what risk factors the cases have been exposed to that those in the control group have not (things like smoking, asbestos, genetic mutations, pollution).

- Researchers then calculate the likelihood (or 'odds') of developing the outcome in people who have been exposed to the risk factors versus those who have not.

Aims: To compare people with and without a specific disease/condition and explain the likelihood of developing this outcome with and without exposure to certain risk factors.

Typical research questions: What factors are associated with an increase or decrease in the outcome of interest?

Real Examples

- Smoking and carcinoma of the lung (Doll and Hill 1950).
- Risk factors for hospital-acquired *Clostridium difficile* infection among paediatric patients with cancer (Daida et al. 2017).
- Stroke in young adults, stroke types and risk factors (Namaganda et al. 2022).
- Association between electronic cigarette use and myocardial infarction (Alzahrani et al. 2018).

Three Unique Design Features

1. **Selection of cases**

   Cases are usually quite easy to identify, e.g. people with lung cancer, radiographers with bad backs, physiotherapists off work with stress. Researchers must provide a clear and unambiguous 'definition of the case' to aid in this identification.

   The selection of cases must be undertaken carefully to reduce the risk of recruitment bias (Coggon et al. 2009). For example, if the case–control study wanted to examine cancer due to exposure to asbestos in the work environment but only selected cases who were young, these cases may not have cancer yet because not enough time has elapsed for cancer cells to develop rather than them really being 'cancer free'.

2. **Selection of controls**

   The validity of a case–control study depends on the enrolment of an appropriate comparison group. Comparison cases (or controls) should represent the same population as the cases using the same inclusion–exclusion criteria. There should be no difference in important factors such as age, sex, socioeconomic status, weight, lifestyle factors such as smoking, alcohol intake, diet. If there are differences this may distort (confound) the results (Coggon et al. 2009).

3. **Calculation of odds**

   Calculating odds in a case–control study is a 'measure of association'. What this means is quantifying the relationship between the relative odds of exposure to a risk factor in the cases versus that of the control group. The calculation of odds is called an 'odds ratio (OR)' and tells us how much higher or lower the likelihood of exposure to the risk factor is in the cases versus the control.

   The odds of exposure among the cases is compared to the odds of exposure to the control group. Imagine this expressed as a fraction. When fractions are calculated the results are *close to, greater than, or less than 1.*

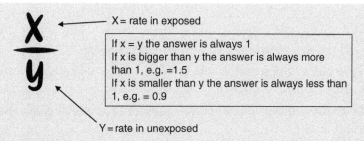

Therefore, where an OR is close to 1 the strength of the association is quite low, but the further away from 1 it is the more likely there is to be a relationship between the exposure and the outcome. For example, an OR of 1.1 does not suggest a strong association. In contrast, an OR of 20 suggests a very strong association. The OR is usually presented with an accompanying confidence level/interval of 95% (see discussion earlier in this chapter). If the confidence interval (the upper and lower values) includes 1, the study must conclude that there is no statistical difference between the groups.

ORs are most commonly reported in case–control studies. However, you may find other results cited. In that case we would recommend reading statistical textbooks like *Statistics at Square One* (Swinscow and Campbell 2002) and *Statistics at Square Two* (Campbell and Jacques 2023).

Strengths

A case–control study is a really useful design to study rare outcomes. They are used when it is unethical or not feasible to expose people to known risk factors (as may be the case in experimental designs), are quicker to conduct, and are cost-effective.

Limitations

Case–control studies cannot establish if the risk factor actually causes the outcome – they can only identify a potential association (or correlation). Case–control studies rely on participants' memory about their exposure to risk factors and may be susceptible to 'recall bias'. If the cases and controls are not selected properly, this can introduce selection bias. Any bias will reduce the validity and generalisability of the findings.

EDECA Appraisal Considerations

Ethics

- Is there appropriate ethical approval/favourable opinion granted for this study?
- Are participants treated fairly?
- What methods in this study were chosen because of ethical principles? Hint – as explained earlier, case–control designs are often chosen when it would be unethical to conduct an experimental design, e.g. it is unethical to withhold a known treatment.

Design

- Why did the researchers choose a case–control design?
- Does the aim of the research reflect what a case–control study can achieve? Hint – case–control studies can only identify association and not causation.
- What are the sources of bias? Hint – look for the possibility of selection bias and recall bias.

Enrol

- How were the cases defined?
- Where were the controls recruited from and are they a good match to the cases? Hint – look for a demographics table showing a statistical comparison between the groups.
- Are there enough participants to be confident in the results? Hint – look for a power calculation or reference to 'statistical power'; anything over 80% is good enough.

Collect

- How are the variables measured and is this done objectively?
- What variables were collected from participants?
- Are there any factors that the researchers did not consider that may have been relevant to the outcome being studied?

Analyse

- What is the magnitude of the odds ratio? Hint – is the OR close to, greater than, or less than 1?
- Are confidence intervals reported and if so, does the figure include the null value (i.e. OR = 1)?
- What is the statistical significance of the exposure being related to the outcome? Hint – look for a small P value, which indicates a lower chance that the association has occurred by chance alone and the greater probability that the exposure is really related to the outcome (Dicker 2018).

Mini Glossary

Cases Group with the outcome of interest.

Control Group without the outcome of interest.

Confounding When an association is identified between the exposure and the outcome but in fact this is caused by something else. Also see the RCT Key Facts Sheet.

Correlation The relationship between two variables, i.e. how changes in one variable are related to changes in another.

Cross-sectional   Collecting one-off data.

Exposure   Any factor associated with the outcome of interest.

Longitudinal   Following up the same sample over a period of time.

Odds ratio   A measure of association between an exposure and an outcome.

Outcome   An event or end point. Also see the RCT Key Facts Sheet.

Retrospective   Methods that look back in time instead of forwards.

Key Resources

Browner, W.S., Newman, T.B., Cummings, S.R., and Grady, D.G. (2022). *Designing Clinical Research*. Philadelphia: Lippincott Williams & Wilkins.

Coggon, D., Rose, G., and Barker, D.J.P. (2003). *Epidemiology for the Uninitiated*. London: BMJ.

Lewallen, S., and Courtright, P. (1998). Epidemiology in practice: case-control studies. *Community Eye Health* 11 (28): 57–58.

Szumilas, M. (2010). Explaining odds ratios. *Journal of the Canadian Academy Psychiatry* 19 (3): 227–229. [Erratum in *Journal of the Canadian Academy Psychiatry* 2015; 24 (1): 58.]

Tenny, S., Kerndt, C.C., and Hoffman, M.R. (2022). Case control studies. In: *StatPearls*. Treasure Island, FL: StatPearls Publishing.

7.4.5   Other Designs

There are some other quantitative research designs that you may want to be aware of such as:

- Case reports.
- Case series.
- (Medical) case studies.

These are reporting types rather than methodologies. These studies generally occupy a low position in a traditional hierarchy of evidence because they do not provide any means of examining causal or correlational relationships. However, they are still very important in providing insight into unique situations or rare conditions. They can be the precursor to a more formal investigation of the problem and they can also alert others to a possible risk or unexpected outcome.

7.5   YOUR TURN!

Now use the blank Key Facts sheet in the Appendix for your chosen study. Once you have completed this, we will show you how to use it to construct your assignment in Chapter 9.

7.6   WRITING ABOUT QUANTITATIVE RESEARCH IN YOUR ASSIGNMENTS

Although you may use this book, the Key Facts sheets, and other resources to make notes about many aspects of your study, when it comes to writing your assignment draft, you should be selective. At level 5 it is important to leave enough room to expand into deeper explanation and analysis, to demonstrate your understanding of the complexities of health research. So this means you will need to be selective about what you present in your assignment. Do not let this put you off making notes – in fact, highlighting quality issues and drafting lots of points means you can 'cherry pick' your best ones, and then refine them further with additional sources and discussion. Remember that you need to show your critical thinking, your wider awareness of research and EBP, and how these connect with the pertinent issues of your study.

General critical thinking about how your study was conducted will make for a strong assignment, but if you can make this specific to the research methodology, then that will enhance your work. So check your points against the four quality markers as you draft, ensure you use some quantitative resources, and look for journal articles or texts related to the specific design that you need to appraise. See the following student examples for some tips on writing up.

7.7   ASSIGNMENT EXAMPLES

Example 1: The study under appraisal is by Anvar et al. (2018) and the aim was to determine the effectiveness of a self-management programme on arthritis symptoms among older women. A quantitative methodology was used, which due to its scientific approach is sometimes considered more accepted than qualitative research (Lakshman et al. 2000). By using numerical data and statistical analysis to answer clinical questions, quantitative research can measure any possible relationship between independent and dependent variables (Elkatawneh 2016; Melnyk and Fineout-Overholt 2019). For Anvar et al.'s (2018) study, the quantitative methodology was appropriate as it could support an investigation of a possible relationship between the self-management programme (independent variable) and arthritis symptoms (dependent variable). However, this methodology is not able to get an in-depth understanding about participants' feelings, experiences, or perceptions (Lakshman et al. 2000; Ellis 2019) of the self-management programme, as qualitative research could have done.

Example 2: Harris et al.'s (2009) study is a randomised controlled trial (RCT) which is a form of quantitative research. RCTs are common in global health research with Collins et al. (2020) recognising them as the most robust design for testing interventions. However, Mulder et al. (2018) suggest RCTs may have a serious limitation in that study populations and conditions often differ to real life.

Randomisation is a key design feature of the RCT, and NICE (2022) explains this as the assigning of participants to different groups without taking any differences or similarities into account. Berger et al. (2021) posit how the basis of any clinical trial involving treatment comparison should be randomisation, helping to mitigate selection bias by giving all participants the same chance of receiving the intervention. Randomisation should thereby increase objectivity and confidence that any difference in results can be attributed to the intervention (Nelson et al. 2015).

7.8 END-OF-CHAPTER CHECKPOINT

		Comment/notes
I can identify the shared characteristics of quantitative methodology	Yes/no	
I can identify a quantitative research question	Yes/no	
I know what data-collection methods are typically used in quantitative designs	Yes/no	
I understand the difference between descriptive and inferential analysis	Yes/no	
I can identify the four quality markers in quantitative research	Yes/no	
I can identify different forms of bias in quantitative research	Yes/no	
I can identify ways researchers can reduce bias in quantitative research	Yes/no	
I can complete the Key Facts sheet for a quantitative study	Yes/no	
On a scale of 1–5, how confident do you feel about the content in this chapter?		

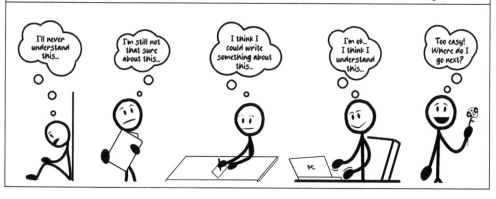

7.9   CHAPTER SUMMARY

In this chapter, we have provided an overview of quantitative research designs including methods that apply to most quantitative studies and those that are design specific. We have introduced you to some key principles underlining quantitative designs, specifically objectivity, validity, reliability, generalisability, and bias (as the overriding concern). You have been provided with Key Facts sheets for surveys, experimental designs, cohort, and case–control studies. In Chapter 9 we will show you how to use the appraisal information to write about your study in an assignment.

REFERENCES

Alzahrani, T., Pena, I., Temesgen, N., and Glantz, S.A. (2018). Association between electronic cigarette use and myocardial infarction. *American Journal of Preventive Medicine* 55 (4): 455–461. https://doi.org/10.1016/j.amepre.2018.05.004.

Anvar, N., Matlabi, H., Safaiyan, A. et al. (2018). Effectiveness of self-management program on arthritis symptoms among older women: a randomized controlled trial study. *Health Care for Women International* 39 (12): 1326–1339. https://doi.org/10.1080/07399332.2018.1438438.

Armitage, J., Bowman, L., Wallendszus, K. et al. (2010). Intensive lowering of LDL cholesterol with 80 mg versus 20 mg simvastatin daily in 12,064 survivors of myocardial infarction: a double-blind randomised trial. *Lancet* 376 (9753): 1658–1659.

Bakker, E.J.M., Kox, J.H.A.M., Miedema, H.S. et al. (2018). Physical and mental determinants of dropout and retention among nursing students: protocol of the SPRiNG cohort study. *BMC Nursing* 17 (1): 27. https://doi.org/10.1186/s12912-018-0296-9.

Barrett, D. and Noble, H. (2019). What are cohort studies? *Evidence-Based Nursing* 22 (4): 95–96. https://doi.org/10.1136/ebnurs-2019-103183.

Beral, V., Hermon, C., Kay, C. et al. (1999). Mortality associated with oral contraceptive use: 25 year follow up of cohort of 46 000 women from Royal College of general practitioners' oral contraception study. *BMJ* 318 (7176): 96–100.

Berger, V.W., Bour, L.J., Carter, K. et al. (2021). Randomization innovative design scientific working group. A roadmap to using randomization in clinical trials. *BMC Medical Research Methodology* 21 (1): 168. https://doi.org/10.1186/s12874-021-01303-z.

Bowling, A. (2002). *Research Methods in Health: Investigating Health and Health Services,* 2e. Maidenhead: Open University Press.

Campbell, M.J. and Jacques, R.M. (2023). *Statistics at Square Two.* Chichester: Wiley.

Coggon, D., Barker, D., and Rose, G. (2009). *Epidemiology for the Uninitiated.* Chichester: Wiley.

Colditz, G.A., Rosner, B.A., and Speizer, F.E. (1996). Risk factors for breast cancer according to family history of breast cancer. *Journal of the National Cancer Institute* 88 (6): 365–371.

Collins, R., Bowman, L., Landray, M., and Peto, R. (2020). The magic of randomization versus the myth of real-world evidence. *New England Journal of Medicine* 674 (8): 382.

Comer, C., Collings, R., McCracken, A. et al. (2022). Allied health professionals' perceptions of research in the United Kingdom national health service: a survey of research capacity and culture. *BMC Health Services Research* 22 (1): 1094. `https://doi.org/10.1186/s12913-022-08465-6`.

Connelly, L.M. and Woolston, W. (2016). Randomized controlled trials. *MEDSURG Nursing* 25 (4): 281.

Coto, J., Restrepo, A., Cejas, I., and Prentiss, S. (2020). The impact of COVID-19 on allied health professions. *PLoS One* 15 (10): e0241328.

Daida, A., Yoshihara, H., Inai, I. et al. (2017). Risk factors for hospital-acquired Clostridium difficile infection among pediatric patients with Cancer. *Journal of Pediatric Hematology/Oncology* 39 (3): e167–e172. `https://doi.org/10.1097/MPH.0000000000000742`.

Deaton, A. and Cartwright, N. (2018). Understanding and misunderstanding randomized controlled trials. *Social Science & Medicine* 210: 2–21.

Dicker, R. (2018). Analyzing and interpreting data. In: *The CDC Field Epidemiology Manual* (ed. S.A. Rasmussen and R.A. Goodman). Oxford University Press `https://www.cdc.gov/eis/field-epi-manual/chapters/analyze-Interpret-Data.html` (accessed 4 December 2023).

Doll, R. and Hill, A.B. (1950). Smoking and carcinoma of the lung; preliminary report. *British Medical Journal* 2 (4682): 739–748. `https://doi.org/10.1136/bmj.2.4682.739`.

Doll, R., Peto, R., Boreham, J., and Sutherland, I. (2000). Smoking and dementia in male British doctors: prospective study. *BMJ* 320 (7242): 1097–1102.

Elkatawneh, H. (2016). Comparing qualitative and quantitative approaches. *Social Science Research Network* `http://dx.doi.org/10.2139/ssrn.2742779`.

Ellis, P. (2019). *Evidence Based Practice in Nursing*. London: Sage.

Harris, N., Lovell, K., Day, J., and Roberts, C. (2009). An evaluation of a medication management training programme for community mental health professionals; service user level outcomes: a cluster randomised controlled trial. *International Journal of Nursing Studies* 46 (5): 645–652.

Hasson, F., McKenna, H., and Keeney, S. (2010). Surveys. In: *The Research Process in Nursing* (ed. K. Gerrish and A. Lacey), 255–266. Chichester: Wiley.

Hill, J., Ziviani, J., Driscoll, C. et al. (2020). Canine assisted occupational therapy for children on the autism spectrum: a pilot randomised control trial. *Journal of Autism and Developmental Disorders* 50: 4106–4120.

Jones, M.K., Weerakoon, P., and Pynor, R.A. (2005). Survey of occupational therapy students' attitudes towards sexual issues in clinical practice. *Occupational Therapy International* 12 (2): 95–106.

Jones, B.P., Tay, E.T., Elikashvili, I. et al. (2016). Feasibility and safety of substituting lung ultrasonography for chest radiography when diagnosing pneumonia in children: a randomized controlled trial. *Chest* 150 (1): 131–138.

Lakshman, M., Sinha, L., Biswas, M. et al. (2000). Quantitative vs qualitative research methods. *Indian Journal of Pediatrics* 67 (5): 369–377. https://doi.org/10.1007/BF02820690.

Madsen, K.M., Hviid, A., Vestergaard, M. et al. (2002). A population-based study of measles, mumps, and rubella vaccination and autism. *New England Journal of Medicine* 347 (19): 1477–1482. https://doi.org/10.1056/NEJMoa021134.

Mann, C.J. (2003). Observational research methods. Research design II: cohort, cross sectional, and case-control studies. *Emergency Medicine Journal* 20 (1): 54–60. https://doi.org/10.1136/emj.20.1.54.

McGough, J.J. and Faraone, S.V. (2009). Estimating the size of treatment effects: moving beyond p values. *Psychiatry (Edgmont)* 6 (10): 21.

Melnyk, B.M. and Fineout-Overholt, E. (2019). *Evidence-Based Practice in Nursing & Healthcare: A Guide to Best Practice*. Philadelphia: Wolters Kluwer.

Morera, O.F. and Stokes, S.M. (2016). Coefficient α as a measure of test score reliability: review of 3 popular misconceptions. *American Journal of Public Health* 106 (3): 458–461. https://doi.org/10.2105/AJPH.2015.302993.

Mulder, R., Singh, A.B., Hamilton, A. et al. (2018). The limitations of using randomised controlled trials as a basis for developing treatment guidelines. *Evidence-Based Mental Health* 21 (1): 4–6.

Namaganda, P., Nakibuuka, J., Kaddumukasa, M., and Katabira, E. (2022). Stroke in young adults, stroke types and risk factors: a case control study. *BMC Neurology* 22 (1): 335. https://doi.org/10.1186/s12883-022-02853-5.

National Institute for Health and Care Excellence (2022). Glossary. www.nice.org.uk/glossary?letter=r (accessed 4 December 2023).

National Institute for Health and Care Research (2024). *Improving inclusion of under-served groups in clinical research: Guidance from INCLUDE project*. [Online] Available at: https://www.nihr.ac.uk/documents/improving-inclusion-of-under-served-groups-in-clinical-research-guidance-from-include-project/25435#what-is-an-underserved-group (Accessed 19 January 2024).

Nelson, A.E., Dumville, J., and Togerson, D. (2015). Experimental research. In: *Research Process in Nursing*, 7e (ed. K. Gerrish and J. Lathlean), 237–254. Wiley Blackwell: Chichester.

Newton, K., Dumville, J., Briggs, M. et al. (2022). Postoperative packing of perianal abscess cavities (PPAC2): randomized clinical trial. *British Journal of Surgery* 109 (10): 951–957. https://doi.org/10.1093/bjs/znac225.

Pezzullo, J. (2013). *Biostatistics for Dummies*. Chichester: Wiley.

Schafer, T., Wood, S., and Williams, R. (2011). A survey into student nurses' attitudes towards mental illness: implications for nurse training. *Nurse Education Today* 31 (4): 328–332.

Scott, I. and Mazhindu, D. (2014). *Statistics for Healthcare Professionals: An Introduction*. London: Sage.

SEARCH Study Collaborative Group (2007). Study of the effectiveness of additional reductions in cholesterol and homocysteine (SEARCH): characteristics of a randomized trial among 12 064 myocardial infarction survivors. *American Heart Journal* 154 (5): 815–823.

Seman, L.J., DeLuca, C., Jenner, J.L. et al. (1999). Lipoprotein(a)-cholesterol and coronary heart disease in the Framingham heart study. *Clinical Chemistry* 45 (7): 1039–1046.

Setia, M.S. (2016). Methodology series module 1: cohort studies. *Indian Journal of Dermatology* 61 (1): 21–25. https://doi.org/10.4103/0019. . .5154.174011.

Stallman, H.M., Ohan, J.L., and Chiera, B. (2019). Reducing distress in university students: a randomised control trial of two online interventions. *Australian Psychologist* 54 (2): 125–131.

Sullivan, G.M. and Feinn, R. (2012). Using effect size – or why the P value is not enough. *Journal of Graduate Medical Education* 4 (3): 279–282.

Swinscow, T.D.V. and Campbell, M.J. (2002). *Statistics at Square One*. London: BMJ.

Tenny, S., Kerndt, C.C., and Hoffman, M.R. (2017). Case control studies. In: *StatPearls*. Treasure Island, FL: StatPearls Publishing.

Whiffin, C.J., Barnes, D. and Henshaw, L. (2024). Critical Appraisal for Healthcare Students: A practical Guide to Writing Evidence-based Practice Assignments. Wiley Blackwell, Chichester.

Zigmond, A.S. and Snaith, R.P. (1983). The hospital anxiety and depression scale. *Acta Psychiatrica Scandinavica* 67 (6): 361–370.

CHAPTER 8

Appraising Qualitative Research

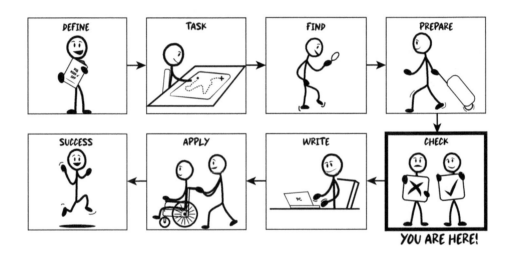

DEFINE • TASK • FIND • PREPARE

SUCCESS • APPLY • WRITE • CHECK

YOU ARE HERE!

FIVE THINGS TO LEARN FROM THIS CHAPTER

1. Qualitative research should not be appraised with the same quality markers as quantitative research.
2. Qualitative research typically aims to develop a rich, authentic understanding of the subjective experience of people and the context in which they live.

Critical Appraisal Skills for Healthcare Students: A Practical Guide to Writing Evidence-based Practice Assignments, First Edition. Charlotte J. Whiffin, Donna Barnes, and Lorraine Henshaw.

3. There are lots of different ways to conduct qualitative research, some of which are more in-depth than others.

4. The main quality markers for appraising qualitative research are subjectivity, credibility, confirmability, and transferability.

5. The overarching concern in qualitative research is reflexivity.

FIVE MINUTES WITH JESSICA, ADULT NURSING STUDENT

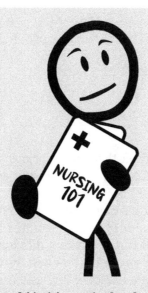

Why did you choose a qualitative study for your assignment?
I chose a qualitative study for my assignment because the subject matter was relevant to my role, and I believed the best way of understanding the issue was through the first-hand experiences of healthcare practitioners. A quantitative study may have been used to provide data that reflected the general consensus and trends on the subject matter; however, it would not provide data reflecting the lived experience from a healthcare practitioner's perspective.

What did you find hardest about appraising your paper?
Understanding the terminology, as this was my first exposure to EBP. I initially found it difficult to get my head around having to appraise a peer-reviewed article, I did not have a clue where to start, but the more I read around qualitative studies and methods, the more I was able to relate and compare to the study. Before I knew it, I was able to critically analyse the methods used by the authors as well as highlighting their flaws within the written article.

What advice do you have for anyone appraising qualitative research?
Question everything that is written within the research. Was it the correct approach? Is there an alternative approach? Which method is best to answer the question?

Read around the research approach, and what methods other authors have used and their rationale. Could it have been applied to the research article you are appraising?

The reading list was very helpful, one of the suggested books contained the information I needed and helped me understand the qualitative approach.

8.1　INTRODUCTION

In this chapter you will be given the general principles of good-quality qualitative research in a similar style to Chapter 7. The chapter ends with Key Facts for several specific qualitative designs.

In Chapter 6 you should have noticed how different qualitative research is to quantitative research. It is because of these differences that the appraisal of qualitative studies needs to be conducted with a different mindset and a different set of quality markers. Therefore, instead of evaluating how a study might have reduced bias (objectivity) and maintained accurate (validity) and consistent (reliability) measurement, and the extent to which the results could be more widely applied (generalisability), other concepts need to be considered.

In this chapter we will explain how to evaluate studies through their ability to obtain the 'insider' perspective (**subjectivity**), their use of robust study methods capable of capturing an authentic representation of the phenomenon under investigation (**credibility**), their demonstration that the findings are based on participant data (**confirmability**), and the degree of resonance that their findings have beyond the study sample (**transferability**).

Aim: To check your familiarity with qualitative terminology

Checkpoint Activity

Instructions: Take a moment to think about subjectivity, credibility, confirmability, and transferability. How familiar do these terms feel? What do you understand by the terms?

It may be helpful to let you know that lots of people find qualitative quality concepts tricky, especially those who are more familiar with the quantitative quality markers, as many working in healthcare are.

8.2   CHARACTERISTICS OF QUALITATIVE RESEARCH

In Chapter 6 you were introduced to the qualitative researcher, their likes and dislikes, and how these apply to research designs. In the *Cochrane Handbook for Systematic Reviews of Interventions*, qualitative research is described simply as 'a research study that uses a qualitative method of data collection *and* analysis' (Noyes et al. 2022). However, it is also worth understanding the difference between 'rich' and 'thin' qualitative research, or some would say big qual versus small qual studies (Braun et al. 2016). Richer qualitative research will provide higher levels of conceptual details, philosophical or theoretical positions that enable researchers to go deeper into the analysis, and will often provide more in-depth understanding of the subject matter under investigation.

Having made a note of this important point, we will describe some of the shared common characteristics of qualitative research (summarised in Table 8.1) and then go on to describe the different types of qualitative research in the Key Facts sheets.

8.2.1   Typical Qualitative Aims

Qualitative studies are usually 'exploratory' or may be 'explanatory'. The researchers should justify the use of these exploratory methods through a research aim that broadly attempts to:

- Describe phenomena, especially those that are not well known, or that occur in populations that have not previously been studied.
- Describe or interpret experience and personal meaning from the perspective of the participant or group.
- Describe or interpret social processes or cultures.
- Generate theory where one does not yet exist.

These aims are often captured by 'what and why' research questions, commonly written as having the following aims:

- To explore.
- To understand.
- To interpret.
- To make sense of.
- To describe.
- To develop theory.

In order to meet these aims of describing, interpreting, or developing theory, qualitative research needs appropriate methods.

TABLE 8.1 Shared characteristics of qualitative research designs.

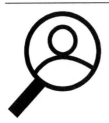

Inside view

Qualitative studies want to get close to the people, groups, cultures, or processes under study.

The insider view is more likely to generate 'rich' findings that fully reflect the nature of that participant's experience and increase understanding of the phenomenon.

Designs are seen as better quality, or more 'credible', if they facilitate a closer relationship between researchers and participants, for example by spending more time with participants.

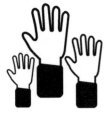

Participant-led research or decreased researcher control

In qualitative research, the participants are considered the experts, so qualitative designs tend to include less structure and manipulation than quantitative designs.

Examples include a more open style of questioning, studies taking place in the participant's natural environment, and sometimes checking findings with the participants before the end of the study.

Methods like this increase the agency of the participant and diminish the power imbalance between researcher and participant.

In some studies participants even work as members of the research team (e.g. co-design).

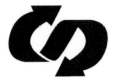

Flexible

Qualitative studies are often very flexible, with stages of the research process overlapping and moving back and forward between stages as the need arises.

This is referred to as an 'iterative' design and it may be necessary when there are unexpected discoveries.

Such discoveries may mean the research team must go back to sample more participants after data analysis has begun, perhaps because it revealed a need for a different perspective.

The benefit of this characteristic is that the research can be responsive to what is emerging from the data, or to the needs of participants.

Assignment Tip

You will demonstrate your understanding of qualitative research better if you apply your explanation of its typical characteristics and aims to the research you are appraising. If you simply describe them, it makes it harder for you to provide any analysis.

Compare these two examples, the first of which is descriptive, the second applied:

- Qualitative research often aims to get an insider perspective on phenomena that have not previously been well-studied (Whiffin et al. 2024).
- Qualitative research often aims to get an insider perspective on phenomena that have not previously been well-studied (Whiffin et al. 2024). This was an appropriate methodology for Smith et al.'s (2020) study*, as they aimed to explore adolescent experiences of vaping cessation, by interviewing teenagers seeking support with quitting or reducing e-cigarette use.

* Smith et al. (2020) is a hypothetical study.

8.2.2 Typical Qualitative Data Collection Methods

The choice of method for a qualitative (or any) study should be led by what is needed to meet the aims of the study. When appraising the methods chosen by qualitative researchers, you should consider how well they enable them to answer their research questions. Typically, qualitative methods include those described in Table 8.2.

8.2.3 Typical Qualitative Samples

Before thinking about the right way to sample in a qualitative study, it is worth remembering what the aim of qualitative research is:

To generate a rich, detailed, and in-depth understanding of the phenomena under investigation.

This aim is quite different to the aim of a quantitative study, which wants to find an answer that can be applied (generalised) to most people. It is therefore unusual for qualitative researchers to achieve, or even aspire to achieve, the sorts of sample sizes that quantitative researchers do. This lack of aspiration for a large sample is driven by a determination to answer the research question in depth, and this usually requires a small sample.

The first time students review a qualitative study their attention is often drawn to the sample size. Students are initially very critical of these small samples and identify

TABLE 8.2 Common qualitative data collection methods.

Qualitative method	What are these?	Why use these?
Interviews	Interviews can be in person, online, or on the telephone.	Interviews are a popular way of collecting information from people. The different styles of interviewing will affect the quality of the data collected.
Semi-structured interviews	Semi-structured means there is a list of questions, but follow-up questions can be added in response to what is said.	Semi-structured interviews are the most common method in qualitative research. They allow the researcher to ask what they want to but to be flexible to incorporate what the participants want to talk about. A common problem is to have too many pre-determined questions that can limit the depth of participant's responses.
Open (unstructured) interviews	Open interviews normally have just one main pre-determined question at the start of the interview and then follow-up questions based on what participants say.	Open interviews put the participant in control of the content of the interview. These work well at getting 'whole stories', but can result in a lot of information not directly related to the research question.
Observations	Watching people go about their normal life Observation can be covert or overt.	Observations are used when the researcher wants to get a view of what happens rather than ask people what they think happens. They are resource intensive, but can lead to a better understanding of culture and context.
Focus groups	Group Interviews with people who share a common experience.	Focus groups are great when you want a collective view on a topic area. However, they can be difficult to manage with lots of people talking. The data obtained can reveal lots of interesting views and shared perspectives that may not have come out in individual interviews.
Diaries	Written account of day-to-day experiences.	Diaries are useful when you want regular updates or data that move through time. Diaries can also be a more reflexive way for participants to contribute to a study. However, they can also be a burden and lots of people do not like writing regularly in this way.
Questionnaire	Open questions where participant's responses are not restricted in any way.	A qualitative questionnaire can be a good way to reach a wider sample. However, people often do not respond to open questions and when they do, they may answer in quite limited ways.

these as a significant limitation. This criticism is exacerbated when the researchers themselves identify the sample size as a limitation in the paper! However, if we accept that generalisability is not the aim and instead qualitative researchers strive for transferability (the degree of resonance that their findings have beyond the study sample), we need to feel more comfortable with smaller samples.

 Research Essentials

Transferability: Transferability can be a difficult concept to grasp. The idea that one person's experience can inform practice and even change practice may, to begin with, seem unlikely. However, in healthcare changing practice based on one event or experience is not uncommon. Think about rare, but critical, incidents and patient feedback. Just because a clinical environment functions really well and 99% of patients report they are satisfied with their care does not mean that this environment should not examine closely the experience of one patient who felt the care provided was not respectful of their cultural needs.

Table 8.3 shows some common approaches to qualitative sampling, all of which have their merits and limitations. Don't forget that appraisal is a balance between the merits and limitations of the choices made by the researcher. Generally qualitative researchers use 'non-random' sampling, meaning that participants are chosen because of what they can tell the researcher about the phenomenon, not because they fully represent the characteristics of the population.

In all studies you need to look at who made it into the final sample. You can then make a judgement about how similar or different the sample is to your clinical context. Here are a few things you may want to look out for:

- Where are the participants from?
- Who was eligible and who wasn't?
- Is the final sample rich in terms of what they know about the subject being investigated?
- What ethical principles may have influenced the way people were recruited to the study?

8.2.4   Typical Qualitative Data Analysis Methods

Once all the data has been collected, it needs to be analysed. Qualitative data analysis is the process of systematically interpreting the data from interview transcripts, observation field notes, or other non-textual materials to develop an authentic

TABLE 8.3　Qualitative sampling methods.

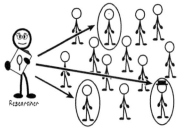

Purposive sampling

Sampling based on specific criteria to identify people who are likely to know a lot about the subject the researchers are investigating

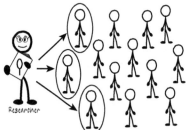

Convenience sampling

Sampling based on recruiting anyone who is available

This is the weakest form of sampling, but often the easiest to recruit

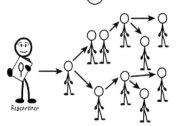

Snowball sampling

Sampling that asks participants to identify other people to take part, so the sample starts small but gets bigger as more people are identified (just like turning a snowball into a snowman)

This is really useful for hard-to-reach groups such as intravenous drug users, or people engaged in controversial activities

description or understanding of the phenomenon – in short, making sense of the data (Wong 2008).

It is typically a long and iterative process, which means it moves back and forth between stages of the research project to accumulate rich data and comprehensive findings. The aim of this iterative process is to ensure that what emerges from the analysis is rooted in the participant data and the context it was collected in. This is not only to improve the quality of the findings, but also to potentially shape later sampling and/or data collection decisions where the research processes of data collection and analysis overlap.

Qualitative analysis is 'deductive' or 'inductive'. **Deductive** analysis starts with theory. This theory can be used as a means of understanding the data or the data collected can be used to confirm if the theory itself is correct or not. In contrast, **inductive** analysis starts from a position of not knowing. The data are instead examined in an exploratory way to discover what it reveals about the issue under investigation. From this examination, a theory may then be developed to help understand the issue.

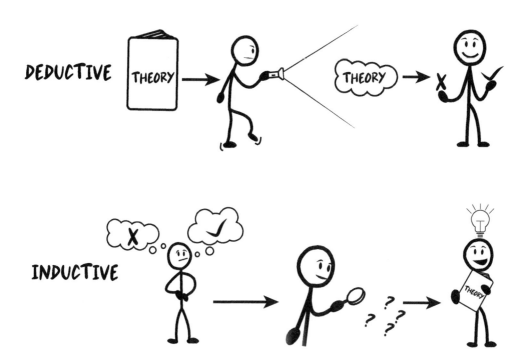

In addition to knowing if analysis is inductive or deductive, it is also important to know if the approach to analysis favours a more descriptive or interpretative style. **Descriptive** analysis stays close to the data and will prioritise the 'who, what, and where of events or experiences' (Kim et al. 2017; Doyle et al. 2020). In contrast, **interpretative** analysis can go beyond what was explicitly said to explore its deeper meaning. In some cases, highly interpretative analysis looks more extensively at what was said and how it was said (Doyle et al. 2020).

 Explore It!

For an example of highly interpretative analysis, look at Elizabeth Stokoe's research using conversation analysis. 'Mothers, single women and sluts: gender, morality and membership categorization in neighbour disputes' (Stokoe 2003) considers how neighbours, as members of the same culture, display their understanding of their identities and activities. An analysis of transcripts from neighbour disputes was conducted with specific attention paid to participants' description of themselves and their description of their neighbour.

In examples like this, it is unlikely that the people from whom the data originated would agree with all the interpretations made by the researcher. Despite this, these are insightful and important studies that reveal hidden biases and subconscious prejudice.

It's crucial for researchers to report what approach and style they used for the data analysis, so that it can be appraised by readers.

 Research Essentials

Deductive analysis starts with theory and uses this within the analytical process.

Inductive analysis starts from the data and works towards generating theory. **Note**: not all qualitative research develops an actual theory.

Descriptive analysis pays more attention to what is explicitly in the data.

Interpretative analysis allows more freedom to explore the meaning of the data.

In addition to the core techniques described here, you should also be able to determine how the analysis was conducted; that is, what steps the researchers took to produce the findings. You may see reference to analysis types like content, thematic, and framework. These share some similarities but differ in their overall analytical approach (see Table 8.4).

TABLE 8.4   Examples of qualitative analysis methods.

Analytical method	Explanation
Thematic analysis	Thematic analysis is an umbrella term for lots of different approaches that lead to themes. Most often a thematic analysis is used to identify meaning, which is achieved by scrutinising the data closely and finding reoccurring patterns of meaning.
Content analysis	Qualitative data are scrutinised for the presence of categories (sometimes these are pre-determined, sometimes not). A content analysis will then examine how often these categories appear in the data as a representation of how important they are.
Framework analysis	Framework analysis uses a pre-existing theory as a 'framework' for what researchers want to look for in the data set. This is a structured approach using a table (called a matrix) to organise all the data. The researcher can then look at all the data that have been put into the framework to help them understand if the pre-existing theory is enough to understand the subject they are exploring, or if they need to advance this theory so it is more reflective of the experiences of people in their study.
Reflexive thematic analysis	A specific approach to thematic analysis that emphasizes the active role of the researcher in creating, understanding and interpreting the data developed by Braun and Clarke (2006, 2019).

TABLE 8.4   (Continued)

Analytical method	Explanation
Constant comparison, open/initial, and axial/focused coding	This approach to analysis is popular because of its systematic approach. Its origins are in a specific type of qualitative research (see Key Facts sheet on grounded theory). Researchers often use this analytical technique in more generic qualitative designs.
Interpretative phenomenological analysis	A specific type of analysis developed by Smith et al. (2009) for a specific type of qualitative research (see Key Facts sheet on phenomenology).
Narrative analysis	Another specific type of analysis usually found in qualitative studies that use narrative inquiry, where the participant's 'story' is analysed for what it reveals about their experience (see Key Facts sheet on narrative inquiry).

The authors of the paper you are reading may or may not tell you the actual steps involved in their analytical work, but if they do not, they should at least indicate where you can find the origin of their approach so you could look up the steps if you wanted to. For instance:

- We used a framework analysis (Gale et al. 2013).
- We used the six stages of Braun and Clarke's (2019) reflexive thematic analysis.

The more detail the better in this section of the paper. Unfortunately, it is not uncommon for researchers to simply report 'we conducted a thematic analysis' and nothing else about the actual steps involved in this process or reference to any analytical theory underpinning their approach. This is poor study reporting – it likens analytical work to a magic trick or pulling the themes out of a hat.

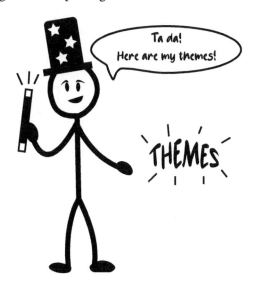

To appraise the analytical method, the paper should report enough detail to show how the researchers moved from the 'raw' data (what the participants said or did) to the final themes, model, or theory.

Detailed reporting of the analysis process is crucial to enable the reader to determine 'confirmability' in relation to the data analysis process. Confirmability relates to how the researchers demonstrate that their interpretation of the data is rooted in the participant data and authentically reflects their experiences of the phenomenon, rather than being driven or selected by the research team (Korstjens and Moser 2018).

But how do researchers 'confirm' that this is the case? There are three main strategies that can be used, outlined in Table 8.5. However, not everyone agrees with these strategies, so we have also summarised the key counterarguments to their use in some qualitative approaches.

8.2.5   Typical Qualitative Findings

Most commonly qualitative research findings are presented as themes with subthemes, or superordinate themes with subordinate themes. For example, Burgess et al. (2021) aimed to examine the experiences of people with mild to moderate dementia, their family carers, and occupational therapists (OTs) of taking part a community OT intervention. One of Burgess et al.'s (2021) themes and the subthemes are presented in Table 8.6.

There are other ways to present findings, such as theories and explanatory models, stories or narratives, and a range of creative techniques such as art-based research, music, sculpture, dance, and pictorial narrative mapping (Lapum et al. 2015; Thompson 2021).

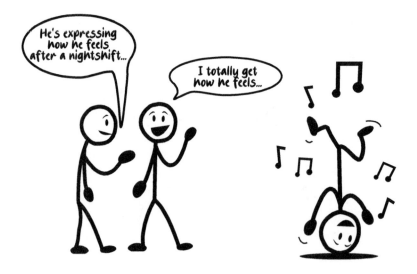

8.2.6   Examples

You can now see how the characteristics of qualitative research play out in the following two examples.

TABLE 8.5 Strategies used by qualitative researchers to confirm their results.

Strategy	What this means	Discussion
Peer checking	Checking interpretations with other researchers.	Some people would argue that 'checking' interpretation with others should be a vehicle to advance interpretation (to go deeper) rather than to 'check' it is correct. This is because in interpretative analysis there is often more than one way to understand a data set, so these critical discussions are a good way to move beyond superficial understanding, avoid assumptions, and ensure important aspects are not missed.
Member checking	Member checking includes asking participants to check the accuracy of data collected.	Not many people ask participants to check data because this can be too onerous. However, member checking can be helpful to the researcher where the source data is unclear e.g. where the audio is unclear on a recording.
Respondent validation	Respondent validation involves asking participants, or other experts outside of the study, to confirm authentic interpretation.	While respondent validation can be a powerful means of ensuring the data represent the original participant's account, some analytical approaches will want to critically explore hidden meaning, values, biases, etc. The participants may not always be aware of these and so may not agree with the interpretation. In such cases the researcher needs to own the interpretation and be clear about the way in which they have analysed the data.
Verbatim quotes	You may have noticed that qualitative study reports are very lengthy and have many long quotes from participants. These are provided so that readers can see the raw data collected and can compare it with the researchers' descriptions of the themes or theory of the findings to check that there is a fit between the two.	It is not just having lots of raw data in a manuscript that makes it credible. Make sure that participants are evenly represented, e.g. the same participant is not quoted lots of times. Make sure there is balance between the raw data and the interpretation from the researcher about what the data means. Having read the verbatim quotes, would you reach a similar understanding about the subject under investigation?

TABLE 8.6 Example theme and subthemes.

Achieving goals	Identifying potential goals
	Selecting and prioritising
	Writing goals
	Achieving goals – factors that enable/hinder

Source: Burgess et al. (2021) / SAGE Publications.

In the first example by Rouch et al. (2022), you can see in the abstract that the aim is to 'explore' the phenomenon of occupational therapy in primary care. The methods include collecting first-hand experiences by talking with a small number (seven) of occupational therapists in semi-structured interviews. Analysis is explained as a thematic analysis and the findings are subsequently reported as four themes.

Exploring Occupational Therapists' Experiences in US Primary Care Settings: A Qualitative Study

Abstract

Importance: Occupational therapy's scope of practice aligns with the goals of comprehensive primary care set forth by the 2010 Patient Protection and Affordable Care Act (Pub. L. 111–148). To successfully integrate occupational therapy into primary care, we must understand occupational therapy practitioners' experiences in this setting.

Objective: To explore facilitators of, barriers to, and recommendations for integrating occupational therapy into primary care.

Design: A descriptive qualitative design that incorporated semistructured interviews, member checking sessions, and deductive thematic analysis. Interviews were structured to capture occupational therapists' experiences of and recommendations for practicing in primary care.

Setting: Primary care.

Participants: A purposive sample of licensed occupational therapists with at least 6 months primary care experience in the United States.

Results: Seven participants reported 1 to 8 yr of experience in primary care. Four themes emerged that contextualized the experiences of occupational therapists in primary care. The first theme captured the process of gaining entry onto the primary care team. Once structurally embedded on the team, the second and third themes, respectively, captured barriers and facilitators to navigating team-based care and providing patient-centered care. The fourth theme reflected participants' vision and ideas of how to expand reach nationally to promote consistent integration of occupational therapy into primary care.

Conclusion and Relevance: Given the important role of an interprofessional primary care team in improving population health, this study is timely in that it explored occupational therapists' experiences in this emerging practice area.

What This Article Adds: Occupational therapists in this study used their skills, resources, and networks to become part of a primary care team. They indicated that they contributed to positive outcomes through working with patients on self-management, functional problem solving, and behaviour change.

Source: Rouch et al. (2022)/John Wiley & Sons.

In the second example by Halberg et al. (2021), arguably the researchers wanted to 'explore' a more complex phenomenon of the 'hero narrative' during the COVID-19 pandemic. Such research takes a more in-depth approach to data collection. Researchers use 'field work', which means observations in the clinical environment, and then add the further data collection method of focus groups to speak directly with clinical staff about their observations and explore the phenomenon in more detail. They use 'abductive analysis' to find the most logical and useful explanation of phenomena, and the findings provide new insight into the 'hero narrative' and the implications of this view of healthcare workers for healthcare practice.

'We Are Not Heroes – The Flipside of the Hero Narrative Amidst the COVID19-Pandemic: A Danish Hospital Ethnography'

Abstract

Aim: To explore how the media and socially established hero narrative, affected the nursing staff who worked in the frontline during the first round of the COVID19-pandemic.

Background: During the COVID19-pandemic, both media, politicians and the public have supported and cheered on the frontline healthcare workers around the world. We have found the hero narrative to be potentially problematic for both nurses and other healthcare workers. This paper presents an analysis and discussion of the consequences of being proclaimed a hero.

Design: Hospital ethnography including fieldwork and focus groups.

Method: Empirical data was collected in a newly opened COVID19-ward in a university hospital in the urban site of Copenhagen, Denmark. Fieldwork was performed from April until the ward closed in the end of May 2020. Succeeding focus group interviews with nursing staff who worked in the COVID19-ward were conducted in June 2020. The data were abductively analysed.

Results: The nursing staff rejected the hero narrative in ways that show how the hero narrative leads to predefined characteristics, ideas of being invincible and self-sacrificing, knowingly and willingly working in risk, transcending duties and imbodying a boundless identity. Being proclaimed as a hero inhibits important discussions of rights and boundaries.

Conclusion: The hero narrative strips the responsibility of the politicians and imposes it onto the hospitals and the *individual heroic healthcare worker*.

Impact: It is our agenda to show how the hero narrative detaches the connection between the politicians, society and healthcare system despite being a political apparatus. When reassessing contingency plans, it is important to incorporate the experiences from the healthcare workers and include their rights and boundaries. Finally, we urge the media to cover a long-lasting pandemic without having the hero narrative as the reigning filter.

Source: Halberg et al. (2021) / John Wiley & Sons.

Checkpoint Activity

Aim: To reflect on the aims and methods of qualitative research

Instructions: Think for a minute about the first example. Do you understand why this study was conducted using qualitative methods? Do any of the findings from this study resonate with your experiences? What skills, resources, and networks did you use last time you tried to integrate yourself into a care team?

Now think about second example. Do you understand why the researchers felt it necessary to carry out observations and focus groups in this study? Do any of the findings resonate with how you feel about healthcare workers being called 'heroes'?

8.3　TYPICAL QUALITY MARKERS FOR QUALITATIVE RESEARCH

8.3.1　Subjectivity, Credibility, Confirmability, Transferability

One of the frustrations in the appraisal of qualitative research is that not all researchers agree about what the quality criteria should be (as explored in Table 8.7). Some people have even asked if we should apply any quality markers for qualitative research at all (Mays and Pope 2000). This latter position is not very helpful when trying to write an assignment based on the appraisal of qualitative research! So while we acknowledge these debates, it is still important to provide those learning how to use and appraise qualitative research with some key indicators of what might strengthen or limit the quality of qualitative studies.

💡 Assignment Tip

You will demonstrate your understanding of research quality better if you *apply* the quality markers, rather than listing them. Students often worry that they may miss something essential in an assignment and listing important concepts can feel like a way of addressing this. However, listing can only be descriptive and does not show your marker that you actually know what those concepts mean. Consider taking the most pertinent issues from your list and weaving them into separate points through your assignment.

Compare these two examples, the first of which is a descriptive list, the second applied:

- Qualitative research has four main quality markers: subjectivity, credibility, confirmability and transferability (Whiffin et al. 2024).

- Good-quality qualitative research should demonstrate credibility in its methods (Whiffin et al. 2024). Smith et al.'s (2020) study* data collection methods were not only ideal for obtaining an insider perspective, but also were of a long duration and so enabled a strong rapport between the researcher and participants.

* Smith et al. (2020) is a hypothetical study.

Table 8.7 explains the four quality markers introduced earlier in this chapter. This table will be helpful for you to return to when you need a refresher.

TABLE 8.7   Explanation of quality markers in qualitative research.

Quality marker	Think of this as. . .	Explanation
Subjectivity	The 'insider' perspective	Subjectivity is about trying to gain an inside view or understanding of another's perspective, specifically the people, group, or setting under study. Qualitative research that takes a more subjective approach is considered better quality because the findings are more likely to reflect the nature of participants' experiences or the phenomenon.
Credibility	Truthfulness	Credibility is about the robustness of the research process and its ability to capture an authentic description or Meaningful understanding of the phenomenon under study. Strategies such as reflexivity, participating in the study group or setting, and developing strong rapport with participants strengthen the credibility of the study.
Confirmability	Demonstrating authentic representation	Confirmability relates to how the study demonstrates that the data collected and analysed fully represent the perspectives and experiences of the participants, and the phenomenon or the setting under study. It includes strategies such as providing word-for-word participant quotes in the study report and strategies such as peer checking, member checking and respondent validation.
Transferability	Applying the findings beyond the sample to similar groups/ settings	Transferability is the degree to which the findings of a qualitative study resonates to similar participants, groups, or settings. It is similar to generalisability and is strengthened by a sample that represents the target population well. However, it doesn't rely on sample size or statistical estimates, but more on the depth and richness of the data.

Source: Adapted from Korstjens and Moser (2018) and Gerrish and Lathleen (2015).

Aim: To understand quality criteria in qualitative research

Checkpoint Activity

Instructions: We are starting to introduce some tricky concepts, so it is worth taking a moment and thinking about what you understand by these terms. In the spaces that follow write your own definitions of these terms and then compare these with the definitions provided in Table 8.7.

Subjectivity means

· ·

· ·

Credibility means

· ·

· ·

Confirmability means

· ·

· ·

Transferability means

· ·

· ·

In Box 8.1 we show you how to apply these concepts to a real study.

Box 8.1   Quality Markers

'It Should Be the Most Natural Thing in the World': Exploring First-Time Mothers' Breastfeeding Difficulties in the UK Using Audio-diaries and Interviews

A qualitative study is designed to answer the question 'What are the experiences of first-time mothers who find breastfeeding challenging?' The methods include audio-diaries recorded twice daily by the mothers, and semi-structured interviews conducted in the mother's own home. The audio-diaries and interviews represent a form of triangulation (**credibility**), with the diaries allowing for a participant-led account of their experiences to be captured as they unfolded (**subjectivity**), while the subsequent interviews allowed for further reflective exploration of important issues. The analysis follows an established analytical interpretative approach, with key steps detailed and the researchers presenting direct quotes to support their findings in the paper (**confirmability**). The study reports the participant characteristics so that readers can assess if the findings may apply to their own patient population (**transferability**).

Source: Adapted from Williamson et al. (2012).

8.3.2   The Overarching Concern in Qualitative Research: Reflexivity

We are now going to introduce a concept that overlaps with these qualitative quality markers: 'reflexivity'. Reflexivity is a core feature of qualitative research and can be seen as both a strategy for managing the **subjective** nature of qualitative studies and a tool to demonstrate **credibility**. We'll explain more with examples here, and then provide a checkpoint activity to help you apply the concept of reflexivity to an appraisal of a qualitative study.

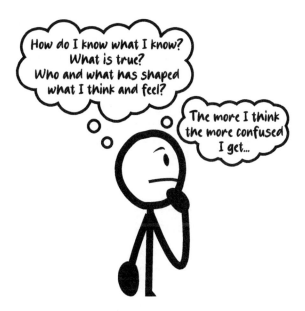

We've established now that qualitative research takes a subjective approach when investigating a topic. This is often by researchers using designs that maximise closeness with participants, or time spent in the study setting, or 'immersing' themselves in the participant data. While these techniques enable the researchers to gain an inside perspective of a phenomenon or an in-depth understanding of another's experience, there is also a risk of the researchers losing their critical or 'research' perspective. Reflexivity provides a way of managing **subjectivity** in a methodical and transparent way. It can prevent the research team from losing sight of the participants' perspectives and can also make clear to readers of the research what influence the researchers' values and experiences may have had on the study findings.

Reflexivity is easier to understand when considered in the context of reflection – a better-recognised technique that as healthcare students you will have been introduced to in the first year of your programmes. **Reflection** is a strategy for learning from our own practice and supports us to develop professional self-awareness. **Reflexivity** goes further, requiring more critical analysis of our values and motives. It is an ongoing process rather than a single act, but the focus on examining personal experiences and contributions to a given situation (in this case, the study) is similar.

 Research Essentials

Reflexivity is understanding the influence the researcher has on the research they have carried out. Qualitative researchers do not have statistical calculations to determine the answers to their research questions. Instead, qualitative researchers must themselves decide what the answer is and are therefore part of the research process.

Reflexivity involves critically reflecting on the position of the researcher and how this has been accounted for in the study. Some considerations will include the researcher's age, gender, and ethnicity; political, religious, and cultural views, socioeconomic status; and personal and professional experiences.

 Checkpoint Activity   **Aim:** To develop insight into the importance of researcher positionality and reflexivity

Instructions: Think for a minute about a study investigating Black men's experience of breast cancer in America. Would it matter if the study was conducted by someone who was white or if they were a woman? Would it matter if the study was conducted by someone who themselves had had a cancer diagnosis? Would it make any difference if the research team lived in England?

There are many different techniques to support reflexivity in research, and we've explained some in Box 8.2. A technique may be used individually, but more commonly a combination will be used throughout the research process. While a study won't report all aspects of reflexivity, it should in theory encompass the entire investigation – from the research team critically analysing their motivations for undertaking the research to how the findings are disseminated and to whom.

Box 8.2   Reflexive Techniques

Reflexive journal

Each researcher keeps a diary as a record of their emotional responses, personal motivations, and reflections during the research process so that they can examine, discuss, and report relevant aspects as the study progresses.

Reflexive memos

This strategy is similar to reflexive journaling, but takes the form of shorter notes made during data collection and analysis. These help the researchers examine their motivations for asking certain questions, ending an interview when they did, or interpreting data in a certain way.

Critical discussions

The previous techniques can aid critical discussions within the team, with research peers outside of the team, and/or with the participants.
These enable the researchers' decision-making to be exposed more widely and be judged by others in terms of the influences on the research process.

Reflexive study reporting

Unlike quantitative research, qualitative studies are reported in a way that acknowledges the contributions of the research team, explains the rationale behind decision-making, and critically discusses how the study and findings were shaped as a result. This is an important hallmark of quality in qualitative research, as it enables readers to appraise how the process was conducted.

Checkpoint Activity

Aim: To locate reflexivity

Instructions: In your qualitative paper, can you find any mention of reflexivity? What other things do you note about the researchers that may have influenced the data? Are the researchers the same or different in any important ways from the population/phenomenon they are studying? Will these similarities or differences add depth/insight generation from this study or detract from it?

Reflexivity is complex and can be tricky for researchers to enact and maintain during studies. However, for students who need to appraise research, the key issues can be summarised by these three points:

- When reading a qualitative study, check if the researchers' personal motivations, relevant experience, or overall position within the study have been discussed and which, if any, strategies have been used to support their reflexivity as researchers.

- Think critically about why the study was conducted in the way it was and if it was reported in sufficient detail for readers like you to judge the potential influence of the researchers on the findings (Barrett et al. 2020).
- If a qualitative study makes no mention of reflexivity and does not appear to discuss the researchers' personal positioning and possible influence on the study, it is fair to evaluate this as impacting negatively on the credibility and overall quality of the research.

8.4   QUALITATIVE DESIGNS KEY FACTS SHEETS

Now you understand quality markers and, more specifically, reflexivity in qualitative research, we are going to look at different qualitative research designs, including qualitative descriptive, phenomenology, grounded theory, ethnography, narrative, and case study designs. Each Key Facts sheet will provide a quick overview of the design, its aims, and typical research questions with some real examples. Three unique design features are then described followed by the EDECA appraisal considerations. A mini glossary is given and some key resources if you want a more advanced understanding.

8.4.1   Qualitative Descriptive Designs

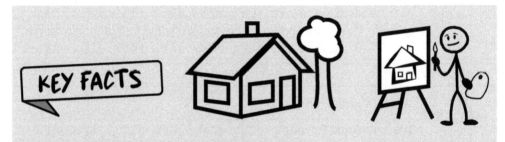

Quick Overview

- Qualitative descriptive designs are often just described as 'qualitative studies', e.g. 'we conducted a qualitative study'. These may also be referred to as generic qualitative or pragmatic qualitative designs.
- Although some descriptive qualitative designs engage in theory to a greater degree for a richer and more complex investigation, typically these studies are more practical. They tend instead to be less driven by theoretical and philo-sophical research traditions and focus on using the methods that best suit the study aim.
- There is debate and some misconceptions around this design, for example that it is, less serious, or makes a less valuable contribution to healthcare

knowledge (Sandelowski 2010). This is related to a lack of published guidance and discussion of its characteristics and a lack of consistency and consensus around its name (Doyle et al. 2020; Kim et al. 2017).

Aim: To comprehensively summarise or describe a phenomenon, event, or experience relating to particular individuals or groups.

Typical research questions/aims: To describe . . .; to explore . . .; to understand . . . Often these questions require a less interpretative approach and are typically used when more specific information is required.

Real Examples

- A qualitative needs assessment of directors of nursing regarding challenges and recommendations for addressing sexual expression and consent (Syme et al. 2016).
- 'Not yet' and 'just ask': barriers and facilitators to advance care planning – a qualitative descriptive study of the perspectives of seriously ill, older patients and their families (Simon et al. 2015).
- Perceptions of cannabis use: a qualitative descriptive study of rheumatology patients (Olson et al. 2023).

Three Unique Design Issues

1. **Focused research questions**

   Kim et al.'s (2017) systematic review examining the characteristics of the qualitative descriptive design found that most studies were focused on exploring participants' experiences, perceptions, knowledge, attitudes, or beliefs in relation to a phenomenon, or its facilitators or challenges. Qualitative descriptive research questions can be relatively narrow or have more boundaries than other qualitative designs and aim to produce a straightforward descriptive account of the phenomenon under study (Doyle et al. 2020).

2. **No strict rules about methods**

   There are no strict rules about method choices in generic qualitative designs. Instead, choices are based on what methods best suit the study aim. Kim et al. (2017) explain that flexibility or variability of methods is a key characteristic of the design and is effective for obtaining rich data and a comprehensive understanding of a phenomenon. Semi-structured interviews are the most commonly used data collection approaches, with focus groups and questionnaires also frequently employed (Doyle et al. 2020).

3. **May 'borrow' methods from other designs**

   Researchers conducting a qualitative descriptive study may 'borrow' elements or techniques from other methodologies or designs (Doyle et al. 2020) but without taking on the related philosophy or full design. For example, a qualitative descriptive study may use grounded theory-influenced data analysis like open and axial coding. Or a narrative-style interviewing technique may be used for data collection, perhaps mixed with ethnographic observation.

Strengths

Qualitative description designs are flexible, specific, practical, pragmatic, and straightforward, and research questions and findings may be more directly relevant to practice.

Limitations

Qualitative description designs can be, but are not always, superficial and ill-defined. They may lack theory, may offer little guidance for researchers, and may be considered 'less credible' than more theoretical or philosophically informed designs.

EDECA: Appraisal Considerations

Ethics

- Was ethical approval/favourable opinion granted for the study?
- Were ethical principles adhered to in terms of consent, confidentiality, risk versus harm?
- What design decisions were made because of ethical principles?

Design

- Do you understand why this design was chosen? Hint – look at the question and how focused/narrow it is.
- Is there any description of theory or philosophy? Hint – look for reference to epistemology, ontology, theoretical or conceptual frameworks. You may see interpretivism, social constructivism, or relativism (see Mini Glossary). If yes, how is this used in the study? If no, does it limit the insights and understanding reached in the research?

Enrol

- What was the final sample size and is this enough to answer the research question? Hint – qualitative descriptive studies can accommodate slightly larger and more diverse samples as the analysis is not always as deep as with other approaches.

- Is anyone missing from the sample that will limit the understanding reached? Hint – check the description of the final sample and think about any under-represented groups in terms of age, sex, race, ethnicity, etc.

Collect

- What justification is there for the data collection methods used and does this seem reasonable?
- Do you think the methods work well to answer the research question?
- Could the methods be improved using a different approach?

Analyse

- Are you told what the analytical process was? Hint – check for reference to thematic analysis, content analysis, constant comparison analysis.
- Do you know why this analysis was chosen? Hint – there are no rules about what should be used in these designs, but they should justify why the approach chosen was the best way.
- Are you clear about what steps were involved in the analysis?
- How confident are you that the findings are a fair representation of what people actually said? Hint – look for strategies like participant validation, peer review, participant validation, member checks.

Mini Glossary

Generic   The research design is not aligned with any established philosophy or theoretical framework.

Member checking   Returning data to participants to check if it accurately reflects their responses.

Pragmatic   Doing what works for the research question and not being overly concerned by philosophical/theoretical influences.

Participant validation   Returning findings to participants for them to check if they agree.

Peer review   Working with other researchers to check, confirm, or advance analysis.

Key Resources

Doyle, L., McCabe, C., Keogh, B. et al. (2020). An overview of the qualitative descriptive design within nursing research. *Journal of Research in Nursing* 25 (5): 443–455.

Kim, H., Sefcik, J.S., and Bradway, C. (2017). Characteristics of qualitative descriptive studies: a systematic review. *Research in Nursing & Health* 40 (1): 23–42.

Lambert, V.A., and Lambert, C.E. (2012). Qualitative descriptive research: an acceptable design. *Pacific Rim International Journal of Nursing Research* 16 (4): 255–256.

Sandelowski, M. (2010). What's in a name? Qualitative description revisited. *Research in Nursing & Health* 33: 77–84.

8.4.2   Phenomenology

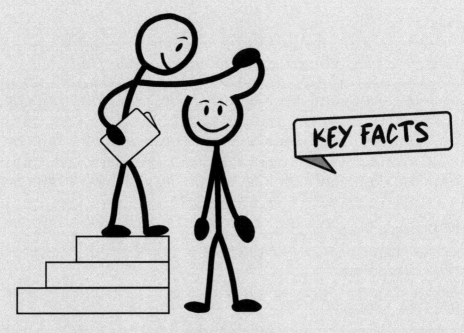

Quick Overview

- Phenomenological research analyses how people consciously experience aspects of life (or 'phenomena') in order to develop a deeper understanding of them (Flood 2010).

- The research design of phenomenology evolved from a branch of eighteenth-century Western philosophy.

- Different types of phenomenological research have now developed, and these can be broadly categorised as 'descriptive phenomenology' and 'hermeneutic or interpretative phenomenology', although in real life there are overlaps between them.

- There are also variations of phenomenology within these two categories, including interpretative phenomenological analysis (IPA) and designs named according to the people who developed the variation, e.g. Colaizzi's, Dahlberg's, or van Manen's approach (Colaizzi 1978; Dahlberg 2006; van Manen 2017). We will only give a general overview of phenomenology here.

Aims: To understand the individual lived experience of a 'phenomenon' and produce an in-depth description, or interpretation, of the meaning attached to it by participants.

Typical research questions/aims: To explore/describe/interpret the lived experience of . . . Questions often focus on understanding the essential features, meanings, or nature of a phenomenon as experienced by a particular group of people within a certain context. Phenomenology should only be used when the research aim requires a much deeper examination of subjective meaning is required.

Real Examples

- The lived experiences of racial bias for Black, Asian and minority ethnic students in practice: a hermeneutic phenomenological study (Pryce-Miller et al. 2023).
- Experiences of adults living with a kidney transplant – effects on physical activity, physical function, and quality of life: a descriptive phenomenological study (Antoun et al. 2022).
- The lived experiences of family members who visit their relatives in Covid-19 intensive care unit for the first time: a phenomenological study (Bartoli et al. 2022).

Three Unique Design Issues

1. **Alignment with the phenomenological philosophical tradition**

   If a phenomenological design has been chosen, the researcher needs to conduct and report the study in a way that demonstrates alignment with its philosophical tradition (or a rationale for why something might have been modified). You should see some discussion of whose philosophical view the research is more aligned to. For example, Edmund Husserl and Martin Heidegger had very different perspectives on how to approach phenomenological inquiry. Husserl advocated a more objective approach whereas Heidegger highlighted the interpretative nature of human experience.

2. **Phenomenological interviews**

   Data collection methods tend to use in-depth interviews, which might be described as phenomenological (Flood 2010) or dialogical (Thomas 2021). This means that rather than being a transactional exchange of question and answer, the participant and the researcher are building an understanding of the phenomenon together through open-ended questions. This is known as 'co-creating' the research findings and it is linked to the qualitative understanding that knowledge, or someone's experience, is not just 'out there' waiting to be discovered and reported. Instead, researchers and participants work together to develop new understanding and any study findings will reflect the input from both as well as the broader context of the interview. Focus groups can also be used in phenomenology, although these are less common. While individual interviews can really facilitate understanding of individual experience, focus groups can aid a more nuanced understanding of social and relational aspects of human experience.

3. **Phenomenological analysis**

Data analysis in phenomenological research can vary significantly depending on the type of phenomenology adopted, particularly in terms of whether a systematic framework is followed step by step, or whether the process is more intuitive. However, you should look for reference to a phenomenological technique such as Giorgi's descriptive phenomenological method (Giorgi 2009), Colaizzi's method of phenomenological data analysis (Colaizzi 1978), or Smith's interpretative phenomenological analysis (Smith et al. 2009). Ultimately, the analysis should provide a set of themes that best represent the essence of the phenomenon, as experienced by participants and interpreted by the researcher.

Strengths

Phenomenology is well established with a strong philosophical basis to develop deep insight. It keeps the person's perception of the issue at the forefront and therefore enables readers to 'walk a mile' in the shoes of the participants (Beck 2021).

Limitations

There is a lack of understanding of and inadequate attention to the philosophical roots of phenomenology and its evolution. It is often used inappropriately when other research designs would be more suitable. There continues to be heated debate about what phenomenology even is and therefore not everyone agrees on the essential quality criteria (Zahavi 2019).

EDECA: Appraisal Considerations

Ethics

- Was ethical approval/favourable opinion granted for the study?
- Were participants aware of the in-depth qualitative approach being used for the study?

Design

- What type of phenomenology does the research state it is? Hint – look for reference to descriptive or interpretative approaches.

- Does the design align well with the aim of the research? Hint – look for reference to the 'lived world' of participants.
- Is there any engagement with phenomenological philosophy?

Enrol

- Can the participants provide meaningful and in-depth insights into the phenomena under investigation?
- Is the sample small enough to facilitate an in-depth analysis?

Collect

- How have the data collection methods been designed to facilitate participants sharing their lived experience?
- Is the data collection conducted for long enough to enable the researcher to understand the 'insider view' of the phenomenon?

Analyse

- Do the researchers uses a phenomenological approach to analysis?
- Do the researchers discuss reflexivity? Hint – look for any discussion of bias, bracketing, assumptions, any characteristics that may influence the way data are analysed, e.g. gender, profession, experience.
- How 'deep' and 'rich' are the themes and subthemes reported in the paper?
- What 'new' knowledge was identified that may not have been revealed through less in-depth qualitative analysis?

Mini Glossary

Bracketing   Researchers try to remove their pre-conceived ideas or theories by 'bracketing' them away so that they can develop more authentic and unbiased research findings (Rodriguez and Smith 2018). This is associated more with descriptive than interpretative phenomenology.

Hermeneutic   Concerned with the interpretation of experience and meaning.

Idiographic   Focusing on an individual's unique perception and understanding.

Lifeworld   The specific social, political, and cultural context that shapes the participants' experience of the phenomenon under study (Flood 2010).

Lived experience   How participants actually feel and understand a phenomenon from the perspective of being in it or having been through it.

Phenomena/phenomenology   Phenomena are just things, facts, or events that can be observed or perceived to exist. So chronic illness, social media use, homelessness, or working in occupational therapy are all examples of phenomena. Phenomenology then, at a very basic level, is the study of whatever phenomenon is of interest.

Key Resources

Dowling, M. (2007). From Husserl to van Manen. A review of different phenomenological approaches. *International Journal of Nursing Studies* 44 (1): 131–142.

Flood, A. (2010). Understanding phenomenology. *Nurse Researcher* 17 (2): 7–15.

Merleau-Ponty, M. (2012). *Phenomenology of Perception*. London: Routledge.

Rodriguez, A., and Smith, J. (2018). Phenomenology as a healthcare research method. *Evidence-Based Nursing* 21 (4): 96–98.

Smith, J.A., Flowers, P., and Larkin, M. (2009). *Interpretative Phenomenological Analysis: Theory, Method, and Research*. London: Sage.

van Manen, M. (1990). *Researching Lived Experience: Human Science for an Action Sensitive Pedagogy*. New York: State University of New York Press.

8.4.3   Grounded Theory

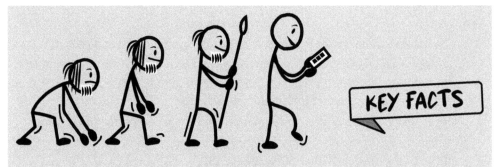

KEY FACTS

Quick Overview

- Grounded theory is one of the most popular qualitative research methods used within the social sciences (McCallin 2003).

- It is an effective way to explore concepts and phenomena relevant for healthcare (Streubert and Carpenter 2011) and for exploring key social processes (Wertz et al. 2011; Charmaz 2014). It is generally used where very little is known about a subject.

- There is often no in-depth literature review at the start of the study. If the researchers do undertake a literature review it is often more like a scoping study and not closely focused on the specific area of inquiry (Dunne 2011).

- Different forms include classical (Glaser and Strauss 1967), evolved (Strauss and Corbin 1990), and constructivist (Charmaz 2006). All forms generate theories that emerge from the analysis of data rather than testing theories through collecting data (Cohen et al. 2011).

- It is important that the theory generated comes from the data not the researchers' preconceived ideas (Charmaz 2014) – hence the term 'grounded' theory.

Aim: To construct a theory that explains or explores the phenomenon (concept/process) being studied informed by the interpretation of participant experience.

Typical research questions/aims: Why do people act/behave/experience phenomena in specific ways? How are experiences made sense of? These questions aim to explore and understand social processes and social contexts.

Real Examples

- The experience of self-care and self-compassion in nursing: a constructivist grounded theory study (Andrews et al. 2020).
- Working through stigma: a constructivist grounded theory of delivering health services to diverse 2SLGBTQ populations (Lane 2023).
- Seeing red: a grounded theory study of women's anger after childbirth (Ou et al. 2022).

Three Unique Design Features

1. **Inductive approach**

   A lot of qualitative research adopts an 'inductive' approach because it generates understanding from the data in the research (i.e. from the ground up) rather than being influenced by pre-existing theory, as may be the case in deductive approaches. However, grounded theory really commits to letting the data do all the talking, even forgoing a literature review in classical grounded theory, so that the analysis is not influenced by what has gone before it. Instead, the researchers engage with related evidence in the analysis phase of their study, incorporating it as data (Dunne 2011).

2. **Iterative data collection and analysis**

   One of the hallmark features of grounded theory is the collection and comparison of data alongside analysis, known as concurrent data collection and constant comparison analysis; these two elements happen side by side (Birks and Mills 2011). This is very different to studies that may collect all their data and then move on to analysis as the next phase in the study. In grounded theory emerging ideas that explain the data are tested out and verified when new data are added. Researchers then look to see if the understanding they have reached changes when new data are added or if it stays the same. This **constant comparison** helps the researcher to move towards a theory that can confidently explain their data set and does not change when new data are added (Sbaraini et al. 2011). This point at which the researchers are confident that their findings are stable is called **theoretical saturation** (Glaser and Strauss 1967).

3. **Generation of theory**

   The process of data collection and analysis eventually culminates in a theory that connects, explains, and incorporates the relationships within the data (Sbaraini et al. 2011). The fundamental aim of grounded theory methodology is to generate substantive theory that can be used to inform future research or inform practice. Importantly, this type of substantive theory is specific to the context of the study only (Birks and Mills 2011). It is through further testing that it can become a more general theory (Charmaz 2014). While other research designs may produce theory, it is not a requirement of their analytical process.

Strengths

Grounded theory is an excellent design to explore concepts where little is known and where theory generation is of benefit to the evidence base. The analysis is systematic and rigorous (this is why researchers often 'borrow' grounded theory analytical techniques without committing to a grounded theory design). The credibility of the theory is increased through techniques such as member checking, triangulation, memo writing (where the researcher notes their thoughts as they analyse), peer debriefing, and reflexivity in the research process.

Limitations

Researchers may not collect enough data to ensure that theoretical saturation is reached. If there is insufficient data, or analysis of the data, the theory generated will be weak or flawed.

EDECA Appraisal Considerations

Ethics

- Is there appropriate ethical approval for this study?
- What decisions did the researchers make based on ethical principles?

Design

- Do they tell you what type of grounded theory they used? Hint – look for reference to 'classical', evolved, or constructivist, or the authors associated with these styles.
- Does the aim of the research complement the specific choice of grounded theory and why?
- Did they review the literature before they collected their data? Hint – classical grounded theory waits until after analysis to review the literature so the analysis is not influenced by prior theory.

Enrol

- How are participants recruited? Hint – look for reference to theoretical sampling, where new participants are recruited because they can provide different views to those already collected.

- How large is the sample given the aim of generating theory? Hint – grounded theory studies can usually accommodate a larger sample because ideally the recruitment should not stop until the researchers have reached data saturation.

Collect

- What do the researchers tell you about the data collection methods?
- Do they use concurrent data collection and analysis techniques?
- How confident are you that these methods have facilitated the researchers' comprehensive exploration of the phenomenon under investigation?

Analyse

- Do they use grounded theory analysis? Hint – look for references to constant comparison or open/axial or initial/focused coding.
- Do they generate a substantive theory and is this theory a good fit for what you know about the subject?
- How did they check their theory was correct? Hint – did they use member checking, peer validation, or triangulation?

Mini Glossary

Concurrent data generation A key tenet of grounded theory, this is what makes it different to other research designs (Birks and Mills 2011). Data generation occurs at the same time as analysis.

Constant comparison analysis The process of comparing newly generated data to all existing data as it arises. When patterns emerge, further generated data is then compared and concepts and categories identified.

Memoing Writing reflexive analytical notes during analysis. This is a core technique in grounded theory, but actually a really useful reflexive strategy in any analysis.

Open/initial and axial/focused coding Open or initial coding is the first step of breaking the data down into units and labelling them with 'codes'. A wide range of codes are often generated first as coding is more exploratory. Axial or focused coding is the next phase where researchers explore relationships and connections between codes to form categories (Sbaraini et al. 2011).

Substantive theory Theory derived from data analysis within a specific, often narrow, research context.

Theoretical sampling A way of selecting participants based on their potential contribution to the emerging theory. Researchers often recruit extra participants to collect data from if they need additional data to explore or verify emerging concepts (Birks and Mills 2011).

Theoretical saturation A point in analysis where no new insights are revealed despite analysing more data. Theoretical saturation is a product of constant comparison and theoretical sampling. However, this term has been borrowed and applied in other types of qualitative research, leading to its overuse and misuse (Saunders et al. 2018). For other qualitative designs that do not use the accompanying methods, data sufficiency (Dey 1999) or information power (Malterud 2001) may be used as an alternative.

Key Resources

Bryant, A., and Charmaz, K. (eds.) (2007). *Doing Grounded Theory: Issues and Discussions*. Thousand Oaks, CA: Sage.

Birks, M., Hoare, K., and Mills, J. (2019). Grounded theory: the FAQs. *International Journal of Qualitative Methods* 18, 1609406919882535.

Birks, M. and Mills, J. (2011). *Grounded Theory: A Practical Guide*. London: Sage.

Charmaz, K. (2006). *Constructing Grounded Theory: A Practical Guide Through Qualitative Analysis*. Thousand Oaks, CA: Sage.

Glaser, B.G., and Strauss, A.L. (1967). *The Discovery of Grounded Theory: Strategies for Qualitative Research*. Chicago: Aldine.

Strauss, A.L., and Corbin, J.M. (1990). *Basics of Qualitative Research: Grounded Theory Procedures and Techniques*. Thousand Oaks, CA: Sage.

8.4.4   Ethnography

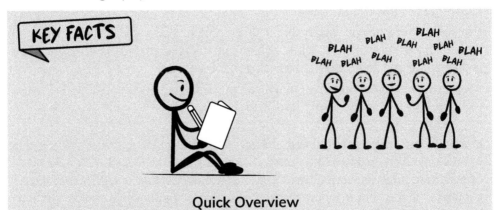

KEY FACTS

Quick Overview

- Ethnography is most used to study cultures, societies, behaviour, and perceptions.
- Ethnography forms the basis of all qualitative inquiry (Morse 2016) and is the foundation of anthropology and sociology.
- There have been many changes to the ethnographic approach over the years as communities, technologies, and knowledge have evolved.
- Historically ethnography sought global understanding of cultures, but now it seeks a more contemporary understanding of specialised subjects (Morse 2016).

- Different types of ethnography are classical, descriptive, critical, auto, and rapid.

Aims: To get 'inside' the way a group of people see the world and to explore complex social or cultural phenomena.

Typical research questions/aims: How does a specific community/societal/environmental culture influence the behaviour, perceptions and/or experiences of the people within it? These questions are typically asked of communities of people.

Real Examples

- Causes of intravenous medication errors: an ethnographic study (Taxis and Barber 2003).
- Communication and relationship dynamics in surgical teams in the operating room: an ethnographic study (Tørring et al. 2019).
- An ethnography of experienced midwives caring for women in labour (Price and Johnson 2006).

Three Unique Design Features

1. **Field research**

   Field research, meaning data collected from the natural environment, is the method most associated with ethnography. In this method the researchers attempt to understand by observing or participating in the everyday activities associated with the phenomenon of interest. Other methods are often added to these observations such as interviews and focus groups as a means of following up, confirming, or challenging what has been observed. The quality of the field work will depend on a number of things such as what the researcher was doing while they were making the observations, how long they were in the setting, and what people knew about why they were there. However, ethnography has been criticised for its 'observer effect'; this is the influence the researcher has on the behaviour of the participants, also known as the Hawthorne effect (Monahan and Fisher 2010).

2. **Ongoing abductive analysis and reflexivity**

   Ethnographers engage in ongoing logical inference and reasoning (adductive analysis) underpinned by critical reflexivity. From observations multiple explanations are examined and tested out. The use of theory is key in developing these explanations as older theories are modified and new theories are developed (Morse 2016). Researcher positionality is also key to how findings are interpreted, so ethnographers must be aware of how and why they interpret data the way they do.

3. **Time**

It should be obvious by now that the methods associated with ethnography take time. Typically, ethnographers spend extended periods of time collecting data (think months and years, rather than weeks). The use of multiple methods also makes for a complex and lengthy analysis. There are additional benefits to prolonged engagement in the field, including a reduction in the Hawthorne effect as the researcher's presence becomes more normalised. However, there is a more contemporary version of ethnography called 'rapid ethnography', which favours a speedier approach to data collection and analysis (Vindrola-Padros 2021).

Strengths

Ethnography offers the ability to attain an insider or 'emic' perspective. It can uncover nuances and social complexities of cultures, promoting a much deeper understanding than other methods can achieve.

Limitations

The researcher can influence the behaviour of the participants. Ethnographic methods are slow to complete. There are often ethical challenges posed by field work, such as observing people without their explicit consent and power hierarchies. While ethnographic studies are very good at understanding specific groups or communities, their findings may lack transferability.

EDECA Appraisal Considerations

Ethics

- Was ethical approval/favourable opinion granted for this study?
- If observations were conducted, were these covert or overt?
- Did everyone who was observed provide explicit consent for this and could they opt out of these observations?

Design

- Are you told what type of ethnography is being used by the researchers?
- Does this type of ethnography suit the research aim and why?

Enrol

- Who were the participants?
- Did the participants reflect the culture under consideration?

Collect

- How immersed in the research setting is the researcher?
- Do the data collection methods facilitate an 'insider view' of the phenomenon being examined?
- How long did the researchers collect data for and do you think this was long enough?

Analyse

- Do the researchers adequately account for how each data type is analysed?
- Do the researchers detail how they combined findings from each data set (this is called triangulation)?
- What is the impact of researcher positionality (see Mini Glossary) on the interpretation of the data?

Mini Glossary

Field work   The practical act of going into an environment to collect data.

Hawthorne effect   The researcher's presence directly influencing someone's behaviour.

Participant observation   Observing people within a community or group and documenting their actions and behaviours.

Prolonged engagement   Spending an extended period of time collecting data to enrich understanding of the research question.

Researcher positionality   Factors that shape how the researcher sees the world and that will influence how they interpret their data.

Triangulation   A method to increase the credibility of a qualitative study by combining theories, methods, or observers.

Key Resources

Atkinson, P., Delamont, S., Coffey, A. et al. (eds.) (2007). *Handbook of Ethnography*. London: Sage.

Fetterman, D.M. (2019). *Ethnography: Step-by-Step*. London: Sage.

Hammersley, M., and Atkinson, P. (1995). *Ethnography: Principles in Practice*, 2e. London: Routledge.

Spradley, J. (1979). *The Ethnographic Interview*. New York: Holt.

Roberts, T. (2009). Understanding ethnography. *British Journal of Midwifery* 17 (5): 291–294.

8.4.5   Narrative Inquiry

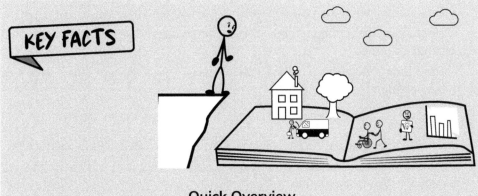

Quick Overview

- Narrative inquiry is best used when there is a need for detailed stories, specific life events, or whole-life histories.
- Narrative inquiry uses storytelling as a means of understanding how someone makes sense of their experience.
- Narrative theory is based on the idea that we know ourselves through the stories we tell.
- Stories can convey the meaning we give to our experiences, through the way characters are cast, how metaphor and imagery are used, how plot lines are developed.
- Narratives can take various forms, including personal anecdotes, life histories, interviews, diaries, or written accounts.

Aims: To understand how people understand their lives through the stories they tell.

Typical research questions/aims: How are stories used to make sense of a specific event or whole life history? How are stories constructed to convey meaning and sense making? Questions are typically broad and exploratory.

Real Examples

- We are not the same people we used to be: an exploration of family biographical narratives and identity change following traumatic brain injury (Whiffin et al. 2019).
- How people with motor neurone disease talk about living with their illness: a narrative study (Brown and Addington-Hall 2008).
- Storylines of ageing with HIV: shifts towards sense making (Beuthin et al. 2015).

Three Unique Design Features

1. **Use of narrative theory**

   Narrative inquiry, as a specific methodology, uses narrative theory to guide both data collection and analysis. Narrative inquiry examines how the retelling of events and experiences in specific ways can reveal more about the experiences than simply identifying a factual account (Bingley et al. 2008). Narrative traditions see people as innate storytellers through which they construct and portray the meaning of their experiences (Lieblich et al. 1998). Stories are always about something, and the way they are crafted reveals something about their meaning. Stories are considered an integral part of our sense of self and our identity. If researchers are using narrative theory to guide the study, you may find them talking about the structure of narratives (e.g. the beginning, middle, and end), temporality, cause and consequence, plot and form, characterisation, and identity construction.

2. **Detailed data collection**

   Participants' stories can be collected in many ways. However, the hallmark of a narrative study is its open and flexible approach to data gathering, which allows the person to confidently tell their story in as much detail as possible. Quite often stories are elicited through a 'grand tour' question that asks the participant to tell their story. This is different to a semi-structured format where participants respond to pre-determined questions. Therefore, look for the unstructured (open) interview method, audio or written diaries, and other forms of unstructured accounts.

   Another strategy to obtain very detailed data is to have a longitudinal design. This method enables the researcher to go back to the participant at another time point. This can be used to see how a story evolves over time, or to ask additional questions about the story following an initial review of the data. These longitudinal methods can increase the credibility of the study.

3. **Narrative analysis**

   A good analytical 'fit' in narrative inquiry is the use of 'narrative analysis'. If using a narrative analysis researchers will attend to the structural and sequential features of an account and should resist fragmenting accounts into simple thematic categories. Narrative analysis may include the exploration of plot lines, characters, metaphor, and imagery. Narrative analytical approaches are the least prescriptive in terms of steps and often researchers must 'build their own' method. This should be deeply reflexive and based on their theoretical framework.

Strengths

Narrative inquiry is participant led, offers deep insights, and is highly reflexive.

Limitations

It may suffer from unfocused data collection, and is resource and time intensive. There is a lack of prescribed analytical steps and the approach requires an experienced researcher/supervisor.

EDECA Appraisal Considerations

Ethics

- Is there ethical approval for this study?
- Are there any ethical concerns about presenting such unique and individual stories?

Design

- How does the study benefit from such an in-depth storied approach?
- Is there a theoretical framework? Hint – studies that are focused on identity construction may use narrative theory as the theoretical framework, while other narrative studies may draw on other theories to shape their methods of data collection and analysis.

Recruit

- Are the participants really 'rich' in terms of their experience and insight into the subject under investigation? Hint – check the inclusion/exclusion criteria, check the final sample description, are participants all very similar or very different?
- Is the sample small enough to facilitate in-depth exploration and interpretation?

Collect

- Do the data collection methods facilitate participants telling 'their' story? Hint – are the methods unstructured?
- How long is given for data collection? Hint – is this long enough to tell their story? Look for evidence of longer interviews such as 60–90 minutes.
- How often do researchers engage with participants? Hint – it may take more than a one-off interview to really get to 'know' a person's story. Therefore, look for ways the researchers have built rapport before data collection or have collected data at more than one point in time (longitudinal).

Analyse

- Do the researchers apply a narrative analysis to the data? Hint – look for ways in which narrative theory has influenced the analysis such as biographical or life stories, structural or Labovian analysis, plot and form (see Mini Glossary).

- Are the findings described as stories or narratives?
- Do the findings have resonance to people outside of the study? Hint – do you find the stories told in this research similar to stories told to you?

Mini Glossary

Autobiographical   A narrative account of an individual's life history told by that person.

Biographical   A study of a single individual's life history.

Chronology   A form of writing that attends to the sequencing of events.

Form   The structure, style, and presentation of the story.

Gestalt   An 'organised whole'. In the context of narrative inquiry, this is the whole story that is more than the sum of its parts.

Labovian narrative analysis   A specific approach to narrative analysis that attends to specific features in the data, namely abstract (what is the story about?); orientation (who, what, and where?); complicating actions (then what happened?); resolution (what happened in the end?); evaluation (so what?); and coda (how does it all end?).

Life history   An extensive account of a person's life.

Longitudinal   A specific research method that involves collecting data from the same person at multiple time points. Longitudinal methods in narrative inquiry provide researchers with a better understanding of the participant's experience.

Narrative   Connecting events into an ordered sequence that has a consequence for later action. The way in which the past, present, and future are ordered creates a 'story' that has meaning.

Plot   Sequencing events or actions to convey the meaning of a story.

Restoration   A way of organising the data in a narrative analysis that creates a beginning, middle, and end.

Storyteller   The person sharing their personal experience.

Structural analysis   Analysis that attends to the organisation of narratives and how the underlying structure reveals how meaning is conveyed.

Temporality   The concept of time, the way it is experienced, understood, and represented within a story.

Key Resources

Andrews, M., Squire, C., and Tamboukou, M. (eds.) (2013). *Doing Narrative Research*, 2e. London: Sage.

Bingley, A.F., Thomas, C., Brown, J. et al. (2008). Developing narrative research in supportive and palliative care: the focus on illness narratives. *Palliative Medicine* 22 (5): 653–658.

Clandinin, D.J., and Connelly, F.M. (2000). *Narrative Inquiry: Experience and Story in Qualitative Research*. San Francisco: Jossey-Bass.

Creswell, J.W. (2007). *Qualitative Inquiry and Research Design: Choosing Among Five Approaches*, 2e. Thousand Oaks, CA: Sage.

Lieblich, A., Tuval-Mashiach, R., and Zilber, T. (1998). *Narrative Research: Reading, Analysis and Interpretation*. Thousand Oaks, CA: Sage.

Polkinghorne, D.E. (1988). *Narrative Knowing and the Human Sciences*. New York: State University of New York Press.

Riessman, C.K. (2008). *Narrative Methods for the Human Sciences*. London: Sage.

Wengraf, T. (2001). *Qualitative Research Interviewing*. London: Sage.

8.4.6   Case Study

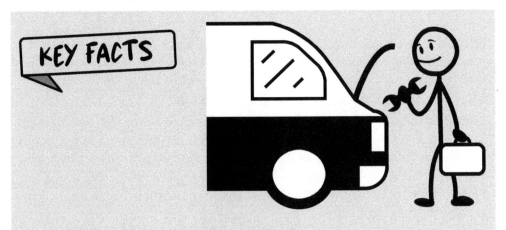

Quick Overview

- Case study methodology gives researchers the means to study a complex system, or systems, taking account of the individual context (Baxter and Jack 2008).

- Case study research is an intense, in-depth analysis of a single unit, situation, or system of interest.

- Case studies are often used to explore complex interconnected, multifaceted research problems (Baxter and Jack 2008).

- Case studies are usually 'multimethod', meaning they collect information from multiple sources. Data collection may be qualitative, quantitative, or mixed (Appleton 2002).

- Robert Yin and Robert Stake are the two most influential authors in case study methodology, but they differ considerably in their approaches (more on this in the unique design features).

- Case studies should not be confused with medical case reports or case series, which are publication types and not qualitative research (Alpi and Evans 2019).

Aims: Case studies take a holistic approach, either selecting a single case of interest and exploring it in depth, or examining multiple cases connected to the same event or phenomenon but perhaps over different settings or groups (Crowe et al. 2011).

Typical research questions/aims: What are the characteristics and features of a specific phenomenon? In what ways are cases similar or different and why? Case study methodology is often used to address questions that need to explain, describe or explore events or circumstances in real-world contexts.

Real Examples

- Implementation and adoption of nationwide electronic health records in secondary care in England: qualitative analysis of interim results from a prospective national evaluation (Robertson et al. 2010).
- Learning about patient safety: organisational context and culture in the education of healthcare professionals (Pearson et al. 2010).

Three Unique Design Issues

1. **Different approaches**

   To understand the use of case study methodology, it is helpful to know whose approach to this form of inquiry is utilised by the researchers and why. In Yin's approach the research design is more aligned to the core values of quantitative research, favouring objectivity and reducing bias. In contrast, Stake's approach is more aligned to the qualitative commitments of subjectivity and reflexivity and more emphasis is placed on the interpretation of data and the social construction of reality.

2. **Case definition**

   For Stake, the case may be intrinsic, instrumental, or collective. Intrinsic cases are selected because they are unique and need to be looked at closely to understand why and how they are so unique. In contrast, the case may be chosen because it is typical of others. These cases can then be studied for what they reveal about the subject of interest (this is called an instrumental design). Collective case studies are used when multiple instrumental cases are identified and comparisons are made between them (Stake 1995). In contrast, for Yin the case may be single or multiple, in addition to being descriptive, exploratory, or explanatory (Appleton 2002).

   In all instances, it is essential that the researchers define what the 'case' is clearly and explicitly before the study is conducted. Sometimes this is quite straightforward. For example, the case may be an organisation or patient group. However, in some situations the case has less defined boundaries, for example the phenomenon being investigated could be 'the decision making-process' or 'care provided by unregistered healthcare workers'. Being clear about the case at the start of the research means the researchers can make informed decisions about what data to collect and who to collect it from to understand the case from multiple perspectives (Baxter and Jack 2008).

3. **Use of multiple methods**

To understand the case in as much detail as possible, case-study approaches usually involve multiple sources of evidence (Appleton 2002). In Yin's approach both quantitative and qualitative data collection methods are used to understand the case. For Stake, qualitative methods are prioritised to reach an in-depth understanding of the case. Quantitative data can still form part of the research design, but the qualitative insights will always lead the understanding that is reached. Case studies can combine data from interviews, focus groups, observations, diaries, patient notes, and many other forms of data. Quantitative methods like questionnaires may also be used. The information gained from these multiple sources of data may be collected concurrently (i.e. at the same time) and then triangulated to reach firmer conclusions about the case under investigation.

Alternatively, the multiple data sources may be collected sequentially, i.e. one after the other where one data set informs the next. You may find the mixed methods Key Facts sheet in the Appendix useful to understand how studies are designed that use multiple forms of data.

Strengths

Using a case study approach results in an in-depth holistic understanding of the problem under investigation. It can provide insight into the sociocultural, political, and organisational factors affecting the case.

Limitations

Case studies can generate too much complex data to analyse in depth. The boundaries may be ill-defined, limiting the insights that are reached. Limited methods will also restrict understanding. The approach may lack generalisation given its focus on single units or a small number of cases.

EDECA Appraisal Considerations

Ethics

- Is there ethical approval for this study?
- Are there any ethical concerns about researching individual cases?

Design

- What type of case study design is being used and is this approach the best way to address the aim of the research question?
- Is the case well defined?

Enrol

- Are the participants the best informants to understand the case and has anyone been missed?
- Is the setting representative of the case under investigation?

Collect

- What are the multiple sources of evidence being used and are these enough to understand the case?
- Could any other data have helped understand the case in more detail/depth?

Analyse

- How have the researchers described the within/between-case analysis?
- What analytical framework has been used to facilitate the analysis of each data set. Hint – each data collection technique will be analysed differently, e.g. interview data may be analysed using a thematic analysis, documents may be analysed using a framework analysis, questionnaire data may be analysed using statistics.
- How has the data from multiple sources been brought together in analysis? Hint – look for reference to triangulation (see Mini Glossary) and how this was achieved.
- Are the analysis methods clearly explained?
- How have they reached their final conclusions about the case(s)?

Mini Glossary

Between-case analysis   Comparison between individual cases to understand how these single units are similar or different. The between-case analysis should facilitate broader conclusions.

Bounded system   The boundaries or limits of the case will define the parameters of the investigation.

Case   The unit of analysis, which can be a single unit or multiple cases.

Intrinsic case study   Focuses on the in-depth examination of a particular case for its own unique qualities.

Instrumental case study   Uses a specific case to gain insight into a broader phenomenon.

Multicase study   Uses multiple cases to gain insight into a broader phenomenon.

Triangulation   Reaching the same conclusion through multiple sources of evidence. **Note**: Some authors advise caution about the assumption that multiple sources of data make a finding 'more true' than if something is only found in one data source. Triangulation will rely on the ways in which the data are collected and interpreted.

Within-case analysis   Analysis of a single case through multiple sources of information (e.g. focus groups, interviews, observations).

Key Resources

Appleton, J.V. (2002). Critiquing approaches to case study design for a constructivist inquiry. *Qualitative Research Journal* 2 (2): 80–97.

Flyvbjerg, B. (2006). Five misunderstandings about case-study research. *Qualitative Inquiry* 12 (2): 219–245.

Merriam, S.B. (2009). *Qualitative Research: A Guide to Design and Implementation*. San Francisco: Jossey-Bass.

Stake, R.E. (1995). *The Art of Case Study Research*. Thousand Oaks, CA: Sage.

Yin, R.K. (2003). *Case Study Research: Design and Methods*, 3e. Thousand Oaks, CA: Sage.

Yin, R.K. (2018). *Case Study Research and Applications: Design and Methods*. Thousand Oaks, CA: Sage.

8.4.7   Other Designs

The Key Facts sheets in this chapter summarise the main approaches to qualitative research. However, there are lots of other methods of which we are unable to provide a detailed review. These include but are not limited to:

- Consensus methods (e.g. Delphi studies).
- Q methodology.
- Participatory research.
- Action research.

If you encounter one of these designs, locate resources that will help you to understand this specific approach before you attempt to appraise it. Having done so, you can complete a Key Facts sheet of your own.

8.5   YOUR TURN!

Now use the blank Key Facts sheet in the Appendix for your chosen study. Once you have completed this, we will show you how to use this to construct your assignment in Chapter 9.

8.6   WRITING ABOUT QUALITATIVE RESEARCH IN YOUR ASSIGNMENT

Although you may use this book, the Key Facts sheets, and other resources to make notes about many aspects of your study when it comes to writing your assignment draft, you should be selective. At level 5 it is important to leave enough room to expand into deeper explanation and analysis, to demonstrate your understanding of the complexities of health research. So this means you will need to choose what to present in your assignment and what to leave out. However, don't let this put you off making lots of notes; in fact, highlighting quality issues and drafting lots of points means you can 'cherry pick' your best ones, and then refine them further with additional sources and discussion. Remember that you need to show your critical thinking, your wider awareness of research and EBP, and how these connect with the pertinent issues of your study.

General critical thinking about how your study was conducted will make for a strong assignment, but if you can keep this is specific to the research methodology, then that will enhance your work. So check your points against the four quality markers as you draft, ensure you use some qualitative resources, and look for journal articles or texts related to the specific design that you need to appraise. See the following student examples for some tips on writing up.

8.7   ASSIGNMENT EXAMPLES

Example 1: The primary study being appraised is by Clayton et al. (2016). It has a clear research aim which is to explore the lived experiences of nurses within a multicultural operating theatre environment. A qualitative research methodology was appropriately used for this aim, as it facilitates understanding behind the lived experience (Ajjawi and Higgs 2007), and attempts to generate answers through direct interaction with the participants (Sullivan and Sargeant 2011). Although close interaction with participants may be considered problematic, Clayton et al. (2016) explain that they use their experiences with participants to interpret and construct an authentic account. Quantitative research and the numerical data it uses, on the other hand, is better suited to explaining trends and measuring relationships between variables (Roni et al. 2020) than exploring social complexities related to communication and experiences (Ajjawi and Higgs 2007).

Example 2: Njogu et al. (2022) used semi-structured interviews and an interview guide, which was developed from the study objectives and a review of relevant literature. According to Ellis (2019), semi-structured interviews are the most used data collection method in health research because they have the advantage of having some structure and prompts, as well as giving an opportunity for the interviewee to offer the thoughts and feelings that they believe to be most pertinent. Although structured interviews have the advantage of following the same protocol, allowing the interviews to be consistent, the closed questioning may generate responses that are not fully developed or sufficiently deep (Ellis 2019) for this type of exploratory study.

To add further credibility to the study, the interview guide was reviewed by a gynaecologist, and a qualitative research expert, as well as being pilot tested prior to the study starting. Having expert reviewers was beneficial because the research team were able to verify the suitability of the interview guide. Conducting a pilot test is also recommended as it enables a check of both interview questions and style, meaning the researcher can be more relaxed and able to generate a good rapport with participants once the study starts (Tod 2015).

8.8   END-OF-CHAPTER CHECKPOINT

		Comment/notes
I can identify the shared characteristics of qualitative methodology	Yes/no	
I can identify a qualitative research question	Yes/no	
I know what data collection methods are typically used in qualitative designs	Yes/no	
I understand the difference between inductive and deductive analysis	Yes/no	
I can identify the four quality markers in qualitative research	Yes/no	
I can identify strategies researchers use to increase confirmability	Yes/no	
I understand the importance of reflexivity to qualitative research	Yes/no	
I can identify ways researchers can demonstrate reflexivity in their research	Yes/no	
I can complete the Key Facts sheet for a qualitative study	Yes/no	

On a scale of 1–5, how confident do you feel about the content in this chapter?

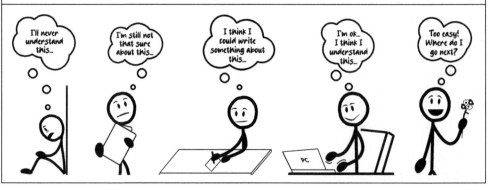

8.9 CHAPTER SUMMARY

In this chapter, we have provided an overview of qualitative research designs, including methods that apply to most qualitative studies and those that are design specific. We have cautioned you not to apply the same quality markers for qualitative research as you do for quantitative research. We have introduced some key terms, including subjectivity, credibility, confirmability, and reflexivity. It is crucial that you understand these in order to appraise qualitative designs. You now have the key facts for a range of specific research designs. In the next chapter we will show you how to use this information to appraise and write about your study in an assignment.

REFERENCES

Ajjawi, R. and Higgs, J. (2007). Using hermeneutic phenomenology to investigate how experienced practitioners learn to communicate clinical reasoning. *Qualitative Report* 12 (4): 612–638. http://dx.doi.org/10.46743/2160-3715/2007.1616.

Alpi, K.M. and Evans, J.J. (2019). Distinguishing case study as a research method from case reports as a publication type. *Journal of the Medical Library Association: JMLA* 107 (1): 1–5. https://doi.org/10.5195/jmla.2019.615.

Andrews, H., Tierney, S., and Seers, K. (2020). Needing permission: the experience of self-care and self-compassion in nursing: a constructivist grounded theory study. *International Journal of Nursing Studies* 101: 103436.

Antoun, J., Brown, D.J., Clarkson, B.G. et al. (2022). Experiences of adults living with a kidney transplant—effects on physical activity, physical function, and quality of life: a descriptive phenomenological study. *Journal of Renal Care* https://doi.org/10.1111/jorc.12443.

Appleton, J.V. (2002). Critiquing approaches to case study design for a constructivist inquiry. *Qualitative Research Journal* 2 (2): 80–97.

Barrett, A., Kajamaa, A., and Johnston, J. (2020). How to... be reflexive when conducting qualitative research. *Clinical Teacher* 17 (1): 9–12. https://doi.org/10.1111/tct.13133.

Bartoli, D., Trotta, F., Pucciarelli, G. et al. (2022). The lived experiences of family members who visit their relatives in Covid-19 intensive care unit for the first time: a phenomenological study. *Heart & Lung* 54: 49–55. https://doi.org/10.1016/j.hrtlng.2022.03.012.

Baxter, P. and Jack, S. (2008). Qualitative case study methodology: study design and implementation for novice researchers. *Qualitative Report* 13 (4): 544–559.

Beck, C.T. (2021). Postpartum onset of panic disorder: a metaphor analysis. *Archives of Psychiatric Nursing* 35 (4): 369–374. https://doi.org/10.1016/j.apnu.2021.05.004.

Beuthin, R.E., Bruce, A., and Sheilds, L. (2015). Storylines of aging with HIV: shifts toward sense making. *Qualitative Health Research* 25 (5): 612–621.

Bingley, A.F., Thomas, C., Brown, J. et al. (2008). Developing narrative research in supportive and palliative care: the focus on illness narratives. *Palliative Medicine* 22 (5): 653–658. https://doi.org/10.1177/0269216308089842.

Birks, M. and Mills, J. (2011). *Grounded Theory: A Practical Guide*. London: Sage.

Braun, V. and Clarke, V. (2006). Using thematic analysis in psychology. *Qualitative Research in Psychology* 3 (2): 77–101. https://doi.org/10.1191/1478088706qp063oa.

Braun, V. and Clarke, V. (2019). Reflecting on reflexive thematic analysis. *Qualitative Research in Sport, Exercise and Health* 11 (4): 589–597. https://doi.org/10.1080/2159676x.2019.1628806.

Braun, V., Clarke, V., and Weate, P. (2016). Using thematic analysis in sport and exercise research. In: *Routledge Handbook of Qualitative Research in Sport and Exercise* (ed. B. Smith and A.C. Sparkes), 589–597. London: Taylor & Francis.

Brown, J. and Addington-Hall, J. (2008). How people with motor neurone disease talk about living with their illness: a narrative study. *Journal of Advanced Nursing* 62 (2): 200–208. https://doi.org/10.1111/j.1365-2648.2007.04588.x.

Burgess, J., Wenborn, J., Di Bona, L. et al. (2021). Taking part in the community occupational therapy in dementia UK intervention from the perspective of people with dementia, family carers and occupational therapists: a qualitative study. *Dementia (London)* 20 (6): 2057–2076. https://doi.org/10.1177/1471301220981240.

Charmaz, K. (2006). *Constructing Grounded Theory: A Practical Guide Through Qualitative Analysis*. London: Sage.

Charmaz, K. (2014). *Constructing Grounded Theory: A Practical Guide Through Qualitative Analysis*, 2e. London: Sage.

Clayton, J., Isaacs, A.N., and Ellender, I. (2016). 'Perioperative nurses' experience of communication. In a multicultural operative theatre: a qualitative study. *International Journal of Nursing Studies* 54 (1): 7–15. http://dx.doi.org/10.1016/j.ijnurstu.2014.02.014.

Cohen, L., Manion, L., and Morrison, K. (2011). *Research Methods in Education*, 7e. London: Routledge.

Colaizzi, P.F. (1978). Psychological research as the phenomenologist views it. In: *Existential-Phenomenological Alternatives for Psychology* (ed. R.S. Valle and M. King), 6. Oxford: Oxford University Press.

Crowe, S., Cresswell, K., Robertson, A. et al. (2011). The case study approach. *BMC Medical Research Methodology* 11 (1): 1–9.

Dahlberg, K. (2006). The essence of essences – the search for meaning structures in phenomenological analysis of lifeworld phenomena. *International Journal of Qualitative Studies on Health and Well-Being* 1 (1): 11–19. https://doi.org/10.1080/17482620500478405.

Dey, I. (1999). *Grounding Grounded Theory: Guidelines for Qualitative Inquiry*. London: Academic Press.

Doyle, L., McCabe, C., Keogh, B. et al. (2020). An overview of the qualitative descriptive design within nursing research. *Journal of Research in Nursing: JRN* 25 (5): 443–455. https://doi.org/10.1177/1744987119880234.

Dunne, C. (2011). The place of the literature review in grounded theory research. *International Journal of Social Research Methodology* 14 (2): 111–124. https://doi.org/10.1080/13645579.2010.494930.

Ellis, P. (2019). *Evidence Based Practice in Nursing*. London: Sage.

Flood, A. (2010). Understanding phenomenology. *Nurse Researcher* 17 (2): 7–15.

Gale, N.K., Heath, G., Cameron, E. et al. (2013). Using the framework method for the analysis of qualitative data in multi-disciplinary health research. *BMC Medical Research Methodology* 13: 117. https://doi.org/10.1186/1471-2288-13-117.

Gerrish, K. and Lathleen, J. (ed.) (2015). *The Research Process in Nursing*, 7e. Chichester: Wiley-Blackwell.

Giorgi, A. (2009). *The Descriptive Phenomenological Method in Psychology: A Modified Husserlian Approach*. Pittsburgh: Duquesne University Press.

Glaser, B.G. and Strauss, A.L. (1967). *The Discovery of Grounded Theory: Strategies for Qualitative Research*. New York: Aldine.

Halberg, N., Jensen, P.S., and Larsen, T.S. (2021). We are not heroes—the flipside of the hero narrative amidst the COVID19-pandemic: a Danish hospital ethnography. *Journal of Advanced Nursing* 77 (5): 2429–2436.

Kim, H., Sefcik, J.S., and Bradway, C. (2017). Characteristics of qualitative descriptive studies: a systematic review. 40 (1): 23–42.

Korstjens, I. and Moser, A. (2018). Series: practical guidance to qualitative research. Part 4: trustworthiness and publishing. *European Journal of General Practice* 24 (1): 120–124. https://doi.org/10.1080/13814788.2017.1375092.

Lane, J. (2023). Working through stigma: a constructivist grounded theory of delivering health services to diverse 2SLGBTQ populations. *Qualitative Health Research* 33 (7): 624–637. https://doi.org/10.1177/10497323231167828.

Lapum, J.L., Liu, L., Hume, S. et al. (2015). Pictorial narrative mapping as a qualitative analytic technique. *International Journal of Qualitative Methods* 14 (5): 1609406915621408. https://doi.org/10.1177/1609406915621408.

Lieblich, A., Tuval-Mashiach, R., and Zilber, T. (1998). *Narrative Research: Reading, Analysis and Interpretation*. Thousand Oaks, CA: Sage.

Malterud, K. (2001). Qualitative research: standards, challenges, and guidelines. *Lancet* 358 (9280): 483–488. https://doi.org/10.1016/S0140-6736(01)05627-6.

van Manen, M. (2017). Phenomenology in its original sense. *Qualitative Health Research* 27 (6): 810–825. https://doi.org/10.1177/1049732317699381.

Mays, N. and Pope, C. (2000). Qualitative research in health care. Assessing quality in qualitative research. *BMJ (Clinical Research Ed.)* 320 (7226): 50–52. https://doi.org/10.1136/bmj.320.7226.50.

McCallin, A.M. (2003). Designing a grounded theory study: some practicalities. *Nursing in Critical Care* 8 (5): 203–208. https://doi.org/10.1046/j.1362-1017.2003.00033.x.

Monahan, T. and Fisher, J.A. (2010). Benefits of 'observer effects': lessons from the field. *Qualitative Research* 10 (3): 357–376.

Morse, J.M. (2016). Underlying ethnography. *Qualitative Health Research* 26 (7): 875–876.

Njogu, A., Njogu, J., Mutisya, A., and Luo, Y. (2022). Experiences of infertile women pursuing treatment in Kenya: a qualitative study. *BMC Women's Health* 22 (1): 1–17.

Noyes, J., Booth, A., Cargo, M. et al. (2022). Qualitative evidence. In: *Cochrane Handbook for Systematic Reviews of Interventions*. Version 6.3 (ed. J.P.T. Higgins, J. Thomas, J. Chandler, et al.). Chichester: Wiley https://www.training.cochrane.org/handbook.

Olson, J., Brophy, H., Turk, T. et al. (2023). Perceptions of cannabis use: a qualitative descriptive study of rheumatology patients. *Journal of Primary Care & Community Health* 14: 21501319231194974. https://doi.org/10.1177/21501319231194974.

Ou, C.H., Hall, W.A., Rodney, P., and Stremler, R. (2022). Seeing red: a grounded theory study of women's anger after childbirth. *Qualitative Health Research* 32 (12): 1780–1794.

Pearson, P., Steven, A., Howe, A. et al. (2010). Learning about patient safety: organizational context and culture in the education of health care professionals. *Journal of Health Services Research & Policy* 15 (1_suppl): 4–10.

Price, M.R. and Johnson, M. (2006). An ethnography of experienced midwives caring for women in labour. *Evidence-Based Midwifery* 4 (3): 101–107.

Pryce-Miller, M., Bliss, E., Airey, A. et al. (2023). The lived experiences of racial bias for black, Asian and minority ethnic students in practice: a hermeneutic phenomenological study. *Nurse Education in Practice* 66: 103532. https://doi.org/10.1016/j.nepr.2022.103532.

Robertson, A., Cresswell, K., Takian, A. et al. (2010). Implementation and adoption of nationwide electronic health records in secondary care in England: qualitative analysis of interim results from a prospective national evaluation. *BMJ* 341: c4564. https://doi.org/10.1136/bmj.c4564.

Rodriguez, A. and Smith, J. (2018). Phenomenology as a healthcare research method. *Evidence-Based Nursing* 21 (4): 96–98. https://doi.org/10.1136/eb-2018-102990.

Roni, S.M., Merga, M.K., and Morris, J.E. (2020). *Conducting Quantitative Research in Education*. Singapore: Springer.

Rouch, S.A., Klinedinst, T.C., White, J.S., and Leland, N.E. (2022). 'Exploring occupational therapists' experiences in U.S. primary care settings: a qualitative study. *American Journal of Occupational Therapy* 76 (1): 7601180010. https://doi.org/10.5014/ajot.2022.049001.

Sandelowski, M. (2010). What's in a name? Qualitative description revisited. *Research in Nursing & Health* 33: 77–84.

Saunders, B., Sim, J., Kingstone, T. et al. (2018). Saturation in qualitative research: exploring its conceptualization and operationalization. *Quality and Quantity* 52 (4): 1893–1907. https://doi.org/10.1007/s11135-017-0574-8.

Sbaraini, A., Carter, S.M., Evans, R.W., and Blinkhorn, A. (2011). How to do a grounded theory study: a worked example of a study of dental practices. *BMC Medical Research Methodology* 11 (1): 128.

Simon, J., Porterfield, P., Bouchal, S.R., and Heyland, D. (2015). 'Not yet' and 'just ask': barriers and facilitators to advance care planning—a qualitative descriptive study of the perspectives of seriously ill, older patients and their families. *BMJ Supportive & Palliative Care* 5 (1): 54–62. https://doi.org/10.1136/bmjspcare-2013-000487.

Smith, J.A., Flowers, P., and Larkin, M.H. (2009). *Interpretative Phenomenological Analysis: Theory, Method and Research*. Los Angeles: Sage.

Stake, R.E. (1995). *The Art of Case Study Research*. Thousand Oaks, CA: Sage.

Stokoe, E.H. (2003). Mothers, single women and sluts: gender, morality and membership categorization in neighbour disputes. *Feminism & Psychology* 13 (3): 317–344. https://doi.org/10.1177/0959353503013003006.

Strauss, A.L. and Corbin, J.M. (1990). *Basics of Qualitative Research: Grounded Theory Procedures and Techniques*. Newbury Park, CA: Sage.

Streubert, H.J. and Carpenter, D.R. (2011). *Qualitative Research in Nursing: Advancing the Humanistic Imperative*. Philadelphia: Wolters Kluwer.

Sullivan, G.M. and Sargeant, J. (2011). Qualities of qualitative research: part 1. *Journal of Graduate Medical Education* 3 (4): 449–452. https://doi.org/10.4300%2FJGME-D-11-00221.1.

Syme, M.L., Lichtenberg, P., and Moye, J. (2016). Recommendations for sexual expression management in long-term care: a qualitative needs assessment. *Journal of Advanced Nursing* 72 (10): 2457–2467. https://doi.org/10.1111/jan.13005.

Taxis, K. and Barber, N. (2003). Causes of intravenous medication errors: an ethnographic study. *BMJ Quality & Safety* 12 (5): 343–347.

Thomas, S.P. (2021). Resolving tensions in phenomenological research interviewing. *Journal of Advanced Nursing* 77 (1): 484–491. https://doi.org/10.1111/jan.14597.

Thompson, M. (2021). Narrative mapping: participant-generated visual methodology for health communication research and pedagogy. *Health Communication* 36 (5): 630–638. https://doi.org/10.1080/10410236.2020.1733228.

Tod, A. (2015). Interviewing. In: *Research Process in Nursing*, 7e (ed. K. Gerrish and J. Lathlean), 387–499. Chichester: Wiley Blackwell.

Tørring, B. et al. (2019). Communication and relationship dynamics in surgical teams in the operating room: an ethnographic study. *BMC Health Services Research* 19: 1–16.

Vindrola-Padros, C. (2021). *Rapid Ethnographies: A Practical Guide*. Cambridge: Cambridge University Press.

Wertz, F.J., McSpadden, E., Charmaz, K. et al. (2011). *Five Ways of Doing Qualitative Analysis: Phenomenological Psychology, Grounded Theory, Discourse Analysis, Narrative Research, and Intuitive Inquiry*. New York: Guilford Press.

Whiffin, C.J., Barnes, D., and Henshaw, L. (2024). *Critical Appraisal Skills for Healthcare Students: A Practical Guide to Writing Evidence-based Practice Assignments.* Chichester: Wiley.

Whiffin, C.J., Ellis-Hill, C., Bailey, C. et al. (2019). We are not the same people we used to be: an exploration of family biographical narratives and identity change following traumatic brain injury. *Neuropsychological Rehabilitation* 29 (8): 1256–1272. https://doi.org/10.1080/09602011.2017.1387577.

Williamson, I., Leeming, D., Lyttle, S., and Johnson, S. (2012). 'It should be the most natural thing in the world': exploring first-time mothers' breastfeeding difficulties in the UK using audio-diaries and interviews. *Maternal & Child Nutrition* 8 (4): 434–447. https://doi.org/10.1111/j.1740-8709.2011.00328.x.

Wong, L. (2008). Data analysis in qualitative research: a brief guide to using Nvivo. *Malaysian Family Physician* 3 (1): 14–20.

Yin, R.K. (2009). *Case Study Research: Design and Methods.* Thousand Oaks, CA: Sage.

Zahavi, D. (2019). Getting it quite wrong: Van Manen and Smith on phenomenology. *Qualitative Health Research* 29 (6): 900–907.

CHAPTER 9

Writing Up Your Research Appraisal

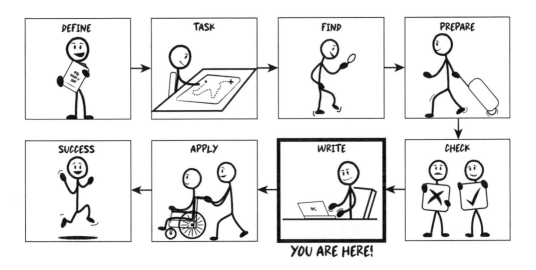

FIVE THINGS TO LEARN FROM THIS CHAPTER

1. Descriptive writing tends to identify issues and state objective information.
2. For appraisal assignments, it is not enough just to describe what a study aimed to do, how it was conducted, and what it found.

Critical Appraisal Skills for Healthcare Students: A Practical Guide to Writing Evidence-based Practice Assignments, First Edition. Charlotte J. Whiffin, Donna Barnes, and Lorraine Henshaw.
© 2024 John Wiley & Sons Ltd. Published 2024 by John Wiley & Sons Ltd.

3. For academic level 5, you instead need to build on this description and create an analysis of the key issues.

4. For appraisal assignments, the analysis takes the form of evaluating the strengths and limitations of the study methods, discussing how they related to research quality, or judging applicability to practice.

5. Breaking down your writing into descriptive and analytical components will improve your writing – this chapter encourages you to try our **Describe-Evaluate-Justify-Support (DJES) tool** to help you achieve just that.

FIVE MINUTES WITH ASHA, PARAMEDIC STUDENT

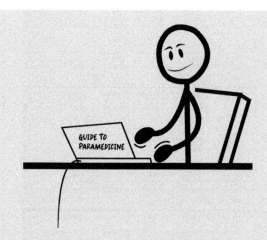

How did you develop a more analytical writing style?
I find it helpful to begin with reading about the issue and then finding at least two sources. Then I start my point by writing 'Such and Such states...' and I build my argument from that. Obviously, you need to have some idea to start the process, to know what to read about and investigate. For example, I might think, 'OK I am going to investigate about data collection in qualitative research'. So I will go and read two or three sources about that and make some notes. Then I've got an idea of what others think, I can apply that to my study and argue for or against that. It gives you a good place to start from.

    I know that others do it the other way round. They start by writing their ideas and then search for sources to support that idea. I did try that once but it didn't work for me. Sometimes you can't find anyone to support your idea and sometimes you spend so long looking that it's just not time efficient.

What did you find the most challenging about writing your appraisal ideas into an essay format?

I think getting to grips with using the language was the hardest thing. Firstly understanding and remembering what the new terminology means. But also using the terminology in your assignment. At first I found it really difficult, but now that I am doing my dissertation I am really enjoying it because I feel I have good foundations of knowing what the key concepts and the key quality issues are.

Getting more confident with the language requires a lot of reading around and that is the other challenging thing. It's very time-consuming to do so much reading around the subject, but it is necessary to help you understand and become familiar with the language and to make your points more informed.

Writing is hard especially when you have placements or work and a family. Fitting in all the reading is difficult and having to keep drafting to make it clear.

What helped you in the writing process?

I normally have issues structuring my essays, but fortunately with this assignment the structure was provided by the research study itself. I was able to support or critically analyse what the authors had written, and used their work to structure my essay.

What feedback did you get from the marker and how do you feel about that now?

The feedback I received was very unexpected but very much appreciated. I put a lot of hard work into the assignment and was relieved that I passed, particularly as we had been pre-warned that the unit was going to be difficult during the early weeks.

Sometimes I've had feedback that I could be more concise. Sometimes I've tried to over-complicate things and the feedback has been to go back to the fundamentals, which is helpful.

What advice would you give to others about the writing process?

My advice would be to plan ahead and make time to read around, perhaps more than you have done previously. I would also say that you should pick a topic or a study that you are really interested in so that it motivates you to put in the time to do the reading and the writing, and it helps you to stay with it.

Use smaller sentences and more paragraphs for flow. Don't use the same reference more than three times!

9.1   INTRODUCTION

The previous chapters have helped you develop your understanding of the typical strategies used for the methodology and design of the study you are appraising. This means you have been able to start scrutinising your study to see aspects of quality, possible limitations, issues affecting who the study could be applied to, or how the findings could be practically used.

Now you need to be able to turn all those critical ideas and notes on the different aspects of your study into an assignment. This is often the part that students find the most difficult because it involves two different challenges: first, understanding the research methods and quality issues of the study well enough to explain them in writing; and second, writing up their ideas in a way that is appropriate for academic level 5.

This chapter will help you to understand what is expected of academic level 5 writing and to notice the difference between descriptive and analytical writing. Descriptive writing tends to identify issues, make statements, and provide some explanation. Analytical writing builds on this, to discuss in more depth *how or why* the issue being identified is important and to provide some interpretation or judgement. It can be hard to grasp the difference between the two in your own writing and to know when you are expanding beyond descriptive writing into analysis, and when you are providing enough analysis. This chapter will provide you with a strategy for identifying the different types of writing and for constructing analytical points for your critical appraisal assignments.

9.2   WRITING ANALYTICALLY

Regardless of what UK higher education setting you are in, the expectations for work at the different academic levels are the same. They are set by the Quality Assurance Agency for Higher Education (QAA), which is the body that maintains and enhances quality and standards in the UK. For qualifications awarded at academic level 5, students are expected to demonstrate critical understanding of their field of study and be able to analyse and interpret information (see Box 9.1 for further details). If you are going on to academic level 6 study, then expectations are that more complex sources of information can be critically analysed and applied, and that understanding of the elements previously mentioned is more advanced.

It is clear, then, that EBP skills of locating, understanding, appraising, and applying different types of evidence is important not only for research modules, but also for higher education programmes more generally. The difference with research assignments is that you are more explicitly focused on the issues of research methods, quality, and applicability and need to show your understanding of these as well as writing about them in a way that demonstrates your ability to critically analyse and apply them to your healthcare field.

Box 9.1   Descriptor for a Higher Education Qualification at Level 5

Foundation degrees are awarded to students who have demonstrated:

- knowledge and critical understanding of the well-established principles of their area(s) of study, and of the way in which those principles have developed
- ability to apply underlying concepts and principles outside the context in which they were first studied, including, where appropriate, the application of those principles in an employment context
- knowledge of the main methods of enquiry in the subject(s) relevant to the named award, and ability to evaluate critically the appropriateness of different approaches to solving problems in the field of study
- an understanding of the limits of their knowledge, and how this influences analyses and interpretations based on that knowledge

Typically, holders of the qualification will be able to:

- use a range of established techniques to initiate and undertake critical analysis of information, and to propose solutions to problems arising from that analysis
- effectively communicate information, arguments and analysis in a variety of forms to specialist and non-specialist audiences and deploy key techniques of the discipline effectively
- undertake further training, develop existing skills and acquire new competences that will enable them to assume significant responsibility within organisations.

Source: QAA (2014).

The other factor that makes research assignments tricky is that students often arrive at these modules with little or no experience in reading a research study. It therefore feels hard to work out and accurately describe what a study aimed to do, how it was conducted, and what it found. So students can expend a lot of effort on submitting an assignment that is primarily a *description* of the study, instead of an appraisal of its merits and limitations. Receiving a disappointing grade or feedback that the assignment was 'too descriptive' or 'lacked analysis' can then be confusing and demoralising.

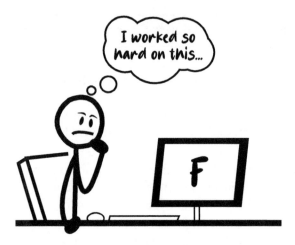

So what can help you to write more analytically in critical appraisal assignments? Being able to identify description *and* analysis; being well informed; and being ready to apply by connecting your appraisal to professional practice.

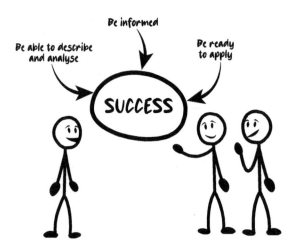

Be able to identify description *and* analysis: The most helpful place to start is by learning to notice the difference between descriptive and analytical writing. Once you've done this, you can then see where you can expand into analysis.

In terms of critical appraisal assignments, descriptive writing tends to be in the form of making statements about the study, for example describing what design or method was used or what the researchers reported. Providing this description is not a bad thing! It is the natural starting point, often giving essential introductory or background information. Without it, your marker would not be able to understand what you were analysing. For example:

- *'The study was a qualitative investigation of the subjective needs of cancer patients waiting for chemotherapy.'*

- *'The study was a randomised controlled trial investigating the use of yoga to reduce the risk of falling in the elderly.'*

Description then needs to be expanded on with your own informed interpretation of why that issue was important to describe. For example, what is that type of design? What types of research questions is it best at answering? What are its limitations? For instance:

- *'A qualitative approach was used because the researchers wanted a more in-depth and subjective understanding of the needs of chemotherapy patients that may not be achievable with a standardised questionnaire because it is not yet known how they feel.'*
- *'The study used a quantitative design because the researchers wanted to measure the differences in rates of falls between those who had participated in a course of yoga and those who do not. Quantitative research is used when an objective approach to answering the research question is required.'*

It can thus be helpful to see descriptive statements as the building blocks to construct your analysis on. Your analysis will build on your description to explain why the information you provided was relevant, applicable, or problematic.

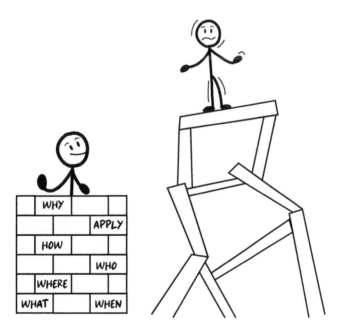

Be informed: To build a strong and accurate point that helps you to achieve your aim of a comprehensive critical appraisal, your analysis should be informed by your wider reading around the topic of research and EBP. Whether that is randomised controlled trial (RCT) design, convenience sampling, or the benefits of using evidence for practice, using the most relevant health research sources will give you the foundations for your analysis. For example:

- *'Only 20 people participated in this study. Small sample sizes are often criticised in research because this can reduce the study's generalisability (Tipton et al. 2016). However, in qualitative studies researchers use small samples to achieve depth in the analysis and reveal understanding that may not be possible had a larger sample participated (Morse 2000).'*
- *'Randomised controlled trials are known as the "gold standard" quantitative design because they are such an effective way to establish causality and reduce bias (Backmann 2017). However, if bias is not controlled these studies are not strong sources of evidence (Mills et al. 2015). In the selected study bias was controlled effectively by blinding participants and using computer randomisation.'*

As with all academic work, using credible sources will enable you to refine the accuracy of your ideas, support them, and expose you to different perspectives on the issue. For EBP-related assignments, it is even more important to demonstrate your ability to consult and use credible evidence.

Be ready to apply: Lastly, being ready to apply your descriptive statements can help you to build an analysis. For students on healthcare programmes, connecting points to relevant issues in practice, the clinical topic, or your professional field more generally is an important way of showing that you understand how the topic relates to your healthcare role. For example:

- *'EBP skills are important as a registrant because they are mandated by the professional body (NMC 2018).'*
- *'This study on staff retention strategies is useful evidence to inform the current debates on safer staffing levels (Shimp 2017).'*

These brief examples start to illustrate the sort of writing expected in level 5 assignments and the important skill of criticality. To help consolidate this writing style we have developed the DJES tool, which uses description, justification, evaluation and support for analytical points in academic writing.

9.3   PREPARING TO WRITE USING THE DJES TOOL

Now you have a better idea of what is expected of level 5 academic writing and how to build analytical writing in a general sense, it's time to put it into practice. We have provided a practical tool to support you to build analytical points relevant to the appraisal of your chosen study. The DJES tool has three main facets – 'describe', 'justify', and 'evaluate' – with a fourth for you to reference your sources.

Describe: Under this heading, simply provide the details from the paper about what the researchers tell you about what they did. For example:

- *'They used focus group interviews.'*
- *'They sent questionnaires to 100 people.'*

Justify: Here, think about *why* the researchers did what they did. Do they provide any justification in the paper? Do you think anything was missing? It might be important to note that here. Even if they do not explicitly justify them, try to consider why they might have made these choices. This stage of thinking critically about your study is really important. You might have some ideas of your own and you can also flick back to Chapter 7 (for quantitative studies) and Chapter 8 (for qualitative studies) for support. For example:

- *'They used semi-structured interviews so that people could talk about other issues the researchers had not planned for.'*
- *'They sent 100 questionnaires because this was everyone who took part in the service they were evaluating.'*

Evaluate: Now think about the strengths and limitations of the design or method you are focused on. Did this technique improve the quality of the study and why? Or could the limitations of the design have impacted on the research findings? Perhaps from your reading around you could suggest an alternative design or method. In terms of an appraisal assignment, this may boost your grades because you are not only providing a comprehensive evaluation of the study but also showing your awareness of a range of research techniques. For example:

- *'Using a focus group method enables the researcher to capture how people respond to what was said which may lead to richer data. However, equally some people may not feel they can express a view that is different from more dominant members of the group. Therefore, in this study individual interviews may have been more appropriate.'*
- *'Only 10% of questionnaires were returned to the researchers. This could mean that the results are not representative because responses from non-responders may differ from those who did.'*

Support: What research or EBP-related texts and articles have you used to explore the issues you've thought about in the Justify or Evaluate columns? Noting them here will ensure that you remember to cite them in your assignment and list them in your reference list. For example:

- *'Using a focus group method enables the researcher to capture how people respond to what was said, which may lead to richer data (Polit and Beck 2021).*

However, equally some people may not feel they can express a view that is different from more dominant members of the group (Goodman and Evans 2015). Therefore, in this study individual interviews may have been more appropriate.'

- '*Only 10% of questionnaires were returned to the researchers. This could mean that the results are not representative because responses from non-responders may differ from those who did (Jones and Rattray 2015).'*

9.4　USING DJES TO BUILD ANALYTICAL POINTS

We now provide some examples of how to use the DJES tool to help you develop your own analytical style. We have also provided a blank template in the Appendix for you to photocopy and use for your assignment.

The examples follow our EDECA acronym that we used in each key facts sheet to represent the key elements of a primary study: Ethics, Design, Enrol, Collect, Analyse. Evaluating these five aspects of your study will mean that you can focus on the key issues, rather than trying to cover everything in your assignment. Once you have completed the table for each of the EDECA sections, you will have the foundation on which to build a great appraisal assignment!

Some things to note in these examples:

- You'll see that it's not necessary to cover all details of the study. If you tried to do this, it would inevitably be superficial rather than a deeper analytical discussion. Remember that at level 5, you need to be selective about your content so that you have room to expand into critical discussion.
- Building your appraisal by focusing on one study element at a time can help you to construct deeper and clearer points of evaluation.
- You may have some points in your appraisal that are longer, going into more critical depth or making two points about that study element while others may be briefer. This is fine if you are demonstrating critical depth in some places.
- The examples provided in this chapter are based on real sources and some of them may relate closely to the study you are using, but don't be tempted to paste parts into your assignment. Instead, use these to help you think critically about the study you are appraising and to guide you in terms of how research sources can inform, refine, and support your appraisal ideas.

9.5 EXAMPLES USING DJES

Appraising ETHICS

Study reference: Newton, K., Dumville, J., Briggs, M. et al. (2022). Postoperative packing of perianal abscess cavities (PPAC2): randomized clinical trial. *British Journal of Surgery* 109 (10): 951–957.

Describe ✎ What did they do?	Justify ❓ Why did they do it?	Evaluate ⚖ Why does this matter? How does it strengthen/limit the study?	Support 📖 What sources have informed your points?
The study noted that wound packing after surgery to treat perianal abscesses was common. However, it was often painful for patients and lacked evidence of benefit. They did this trial to test whether or not packing perianal abscess could be as effective for postoperative healing and less painful. In terms of ethics, the researchers briefly note that ethical approval was obtained from an ethics committee and that numerous patients withdrew consent during the study.	Possible limitation: no detail reported on the consent process or how any other ethical issues were managed. This is problematic because the study is on a sensitive and painful physical problem. Also involved participants being randomly allocated to have potentially painful wound-packing procedures. Did they get enough information on the study risks? How were participants' privacy and dignity protected? Possible strength: it was reported that lots of participants withdrew consent, so it seems they didn't feel coerced to continue.	Researchers should report the details of relevant ethical issues and processes so that readers can fully evaluate a study. However, many RCTs fail to report or provide sufficient detail on how participants were informed of the risks/harms of the study, and if consent was checked throughout the study (Ferrarello et al. 2018). Gaining consent for research should involve the researchers providing full and clear information about the potential harms of the study, no direct/indirect coercion, and opportunities for consent to be withdrawn (Gerrish and Lathlean 2015)	Ferrarello, F., Viligiardi, M., and Di Bari, M. (2018). Ethics reporting practices in randomized controlled trials of physical therapy interventions after stroke. *Archives of Physiotherapy* 8: 1–10. Gerrish, K. and Lathlean, J. (2015). *The Research Process in Nursing*, Chichester: Wiley.

(Continued)

An example of using the DJES answers to create an analytical appraisal point

[DESCRIBE] Newton et al.'s (2022) randomised controlled trial aimed to test if non-packing of perianal abscess cavities after surgery is less painful than packing, and if there was any detrimental impact on wound healing in comparison to packing. They reported that ethical approval was obtained from an ethics committee, but no detail on the consent process or any other ethical issues. [JUSTIFY] Relevant ethical issues for this study include the fact that it is a sensitive and painful physical problem and being randomly allocated to have potentially painful wound packing or not. [EVALUATE] Ferrarello et al. (2018) argue that researchers should report the details of relevant ethical issues and processes so the study can be fully evaluated, but that it is common for details relating to the consent process to be missed. A robust consent process should include sufficient and accessible information on the potential harms of the study, no direct or indirect coercion, and opportunities for consent to be withdrawn (Gerrish and Lathlean 2015). [DESCRIBE] On the issue of withdrawal, Newton et al. (2002) did report that many participants dropped out during the study, which [JUSTIFY] suggests they did have the opportunity to do so and did not feel coerced to continue. [EVALUATE] Therefore, while more detail is needed to be reported on consent, privacy, and dignity, it can be argued that participant autonomy to exit the study was protected.

Appraising DESIGN

Study reference: Zemlak, J.L., Alexander, K.A., Wilson, D., and Sherman, S.G. (2023). Contraceptive decision-making through the lens of social determinants of health among female sex workers: a qualitative descriptive study. *Journal of Advanced Nursing* 79: 1898–1911.

Describe ✏️ What did they do?	Justify ❓ Why did they do it?	Evaluate ⚖️ Why does this matter? How does it strengthen/limit the study?	Support 📖 What sources have informed your points?
The study used a qualitative descriptive design to explore how female sex workers make decisions about contraception, with a focus on social determinants of health such as poverty, access to healthcare, and neighbourhood environment.	No clear explanation about why the qualitative descriptive design was chosen. But these designs tend to be used for focused or specific qualitative questions. So it is a good fit with this study's very specific research questions (how social determinants of health influenced sex workers' contraceptive decision-making).	The research question needs to match the chosen research design, otherwise the study may not achieve its aim effectively (Teherani et al. 2015). Qualitative descriptive designs are appropriate for more focused research questions that have a specific objective, and are descriptive (explaining how things are) rather than interpretative (Doyle et al. 2020).	Teherani, A., Martimianakis, T., Stenfors-Hayes, T. et al. (2015). Choosing a qualitative research approach. *Journal of Graduate Medical Education* (4): 669–670. Doyle, L., McCabe, C., Keogh, B. et al. (2020). An overview of the qualitative descriptive design within nursing research. *Journal of Research in Nursing* 25 (5): 443–455.

An example of using the DJES answers to create an analytical appraisal point

[DESCRIBE] Zemlak et al.'s (2023) study used a qualitative descriptive design. [JUSTIFY] The researchers do not report explicitly why they chose this design. [EVALUATE] However, Doyle et al. (2020) explain that focused research questions that have a specific objective are well suited to a qualitative descriptive research design. [JUSTIFY] For this study, the research question was very specific in terms of scope as it set out to examine how social determinants of health influenced sex workers' contraceptive decision-making. The research question must match [EVALUATE] the research design as this can mean that a study is more likely to achieve its objectives (Teherani et al. 2015). Therefore, Zemlak et al.'s (2023) design can be considered appropriate and effective.

Appraising ENROL

Study reference: Bedston, S., Akbari, A., Jarvis, C.I. et al. (2022). COVID-19 vaccine uptake, effectiveness, and waning in 82,959 health care workers: a national prospective cohort study in Wales. *Vaccine* 40 (8): 1180–1189.

Describe 🖉 What did they do?	Justify ❓ Why did they do it?	Evaluate ⚖️ Why does this matter? How does it strengthen/limit the study?	Support 📖 What sources have informed your points?
This was a prospective cohort study to examine COVID-19 and vaccination in Welsh healthcare worker (HCW) populations. To enrol participants, they used a national databank to identify 104 784 potentially eligible HCWs. After excluding those who didn't have full records available and those who had already had COVID-19, they analysed data from 82 959 participants. They didn't report any significant attrition but censored observations for those who died, moved out of healthcare work, or left Wales (4.6%).	Selecting their cohort of participants from a national databank rather than asking participants to volunteer for the study has two possible strengths: a very large sample size was achieved, and the sample was more likely to be representative of the population (in this case, healthcare workers in Wales). However, there may have been some bias related to those who could not be followed up to the end of the study (those who died from a non-COVID-19 cause, moved out of healthcare work, or left Wales). The number of people who could not be followed up to the end point of the study was only 4.6% of the large sample, so this may not have caused a significant limitation.	One of the strengths of cohort studies is that they can draw confident conclusions regarding the link between risk factors and disease across longer time frames than other designs. However, participants may drop out, increasing the risk of attrition bias (Barrett and Noble 2019). In cohort studies the follow-up of participants is very important. If there is large attrition (or drop-out) where participants cannot be followed up then this is a source of bias, especially where the participants dropping out have similar characteristics (e.g. they were identified at baseline as having more severe disease). If the proportion is very high (>30%), then the validity of the results from this study is doubtful (Setia 2016).	Barrett, D., and Noble, H. (2019). What are cohort studies? *Evidence-Based Nursing* 22 (4): 95–96. Gerrish, K., and Lathlean, J. (2015). *The Research Process in Nursing*. Chichester: Wiley. Setia, M.S. (2016). Methodology series module 1: cohort studies. *Indian Journal of Dermatology* 61 (1): 21–25.

An example of using the DJES answers to create an analytical appraisal point

[DESCRIBE] Bedston et al.'s (2022) prospective cohort study used a Welsh national databank to identify 104 784 potentially eligible HCWs. After excluding those without full records and those who had already had COVID-19, they had a sample size of 82 959 participants. They didn't report any significant attrition but censored observations for those who died, moved out of healthcare work, or left Wales (4.6%). [JUSTIFY] By enrolling participants from a national databank, rather than asking participants to volunteer for the study, Bedston et al.'s (2022) study was able to achieve a large sample size that was more likely to be representative of the population (in his case, healthcare workers in Wales). [EVALUATE] Barret and Noble (2019) note that large-scale cohort studies like this are more likely to be able to draw confident conclusions regarding the link between risk factors and disease across longer time frames than other designs.

[EVALUATE] However, there is also a risk that participants may drop out, potentially causing attrition bias (Barrett and Noble 2019), because data can no longer be collected on those who drop out of the study (Setia 2016). [DESCRIBE] Bedston et al. (2022) report that 4.6% of the sample could not be followed up because they either died (from a cause not related to COVID-19), moved out of healthcare work, or left Wales. [EVALUATE] Setia (2016) explains that the validity of the results can be weakened if the participants dropping out have similar characteristics (e.g. they were identified at baseline as having more severe disease) or if the proportion dropping out is very high, for example more than 30% of the sample. [JUSTIFY] It can be argued that as Bedston et al.'s (2022) drop-out was a small proportion of the sample and the reasons were clearly reported and accounted for in the analysis, [EVALUATE] this was not a major limitation of the study.

Appraising COLLECT

Study reference: Pryce-Miller, M., Bliss, E., Airey, A. et al. (2023). The lived experiences of racial bias for black, Asian and minority ethnic students in practice: a hermeneutic phenomenological study. *Nurse Education in Practice* 66: 103532.

Describe ✎ What did they do?	Justify ❓ Why did they do it?	Evaluate ⚖ Why does this matter? How does it strengthen/limit the study?	Support 📖 What sources have informed your points?
This phenomenological study explored the lived experiences of racial bias for Black, Asian, and minority ethnic students undertaking an undergraduate or postgraduate degree in UK nursing, midwifery, and allied health courses. They used two methods of data collection, focus groups (2-hour duration) and individual semi-structured interviews (1-hour duration). Both were conducted online due to the COVID-19 lock-down. The researchers report using a phenomenological interview technique that was conversational and followed a topic guide.	Using two methods might be a stronger way of collecting data, being able to understand the topic from different perspectives. The researchers followed a phenomenological rather than generic style of interview and seem to have conducted the interviews for sufficient time to gain insight and develop a comfortable relationship with the participants, especially as they were discussing a sensitive and potentially distressing subject. Using two different methods might be a way of getting a broader picture of the issue under study.	Interviews in phenomenology should be a 'co-creation' between the researcher and the participant, where both parties are developing insight into the issue under study, and the interviewer is probing and exploring rather than directing the participant (Flood 2010). The use of two different methods to collect data is a form of 'triangulation' that is done so that the researchers can combine findings from two or more rigorous approaches and therefore achieve a more comprehensive set of data overall (Heale and Forbes 2013).	Flood, A. (2010) Understanding phenomenology. *Nurse Researcher* 17 (2). Heale, R., and Forbes, D. (2013). Understanding triangulation in research. *Evidence-Based Nursing* 16 (4): 98–99.

An example of using the DJES answers to create an analytical appraisal point

[DESCRIBE] Pryce-Miller et al. (2023) collected data using two online methods: focus groups lasting 2 hours and individual semi-structured interviews lasting 1 hour. [JUSTIFY] Using two different data collection methods strengthens the study as it allows the researchers to [EVALUATE] combine the data and get a more comprehensive understanding of the topic through a 'triangulation' technique (Health and Forbes 2013).

[DESCRIBE] In terms of the interviews, the researchers detail that these were phenomenological in style, with a conversational manner. [JUSTIFY] They also seemed to have conducted them for sufficient time to gain an 'inside view' and develop a comfortable relationship with the participants, especially as they were discussing a sensitive and potentially distressing subject. [EVALUATE] Flood (2010) notes that the duration and the conversational style give credibility to phenomenological studies as they facilitate a 'co-creation' between the researcher and the participant, with probing and exploring that generate insight into the issue under study.

Appraising ANALYSE

Study reference: Comer, C., Collings, R., McCracken, A. et al. (2022). Allied health professionals' perceptions of research in the United Kingdom national health service: a survey of research capacity and culture. *BMC Health Services Research* 22: 1094. https://doi.org/10.1186/s12913-022-08465-6.

Describe ✏️ What did they do?	Justify ❓ Why did they do it?	Evaluate ⚖️ Why does this matter? How does it strengthen/limit the study?	Support 📖 What sources have informed your points?
The researchers used a descriptive analysis, using aggregate median scores, inter-quartile ranges (IQR), and percentages to describe the results. The main study results were that research success at an individual level was perceived as adequate (median = 4; IQR 2–6), as was that of the organisation (median = 4; IQR 2–7). However, research success as a team was perceived as less than adequate (median score 2; IQR 1–5). Key barriers to research included 'other work roles take priority' (83%) and 'lack of time for research' (80%), whereas motivators included 'to develop skills' (80%) and 'increased job satisfaction' (63%).	The median value is commonly chosen for rank data because the mean is not always appropriate. IQRs are useful to show the variability of responses around the median value, whereas percentages are a good way to show how many people responded in the same way.	Descriptive statistics are an excellent way to describe and summarise the data. Given that the aim of the study was to understand perceptions of research, this approach to analysis seems appropriate. However, it may have been possible to have identified and test hypotheses using inferential statistics to make predictions beyond the immediate study data. This may have improved the generalisability of the study findings.	Sullivan, G.M. and Artino, A.R. (2013). Analyzing and interpreting data from Likert-type scales. *Journal of Graduate Medical Education* 5 (4): 541–542. https://doi.org/10.4300/JGME-5-4-18. Sullivan-Bolyai, S. and Bova, C. (2018). Data analysis: descriptive and inferential statistics. In: LoBiondo-Wood, G. and Haber, J. (eds.) *Nursing Research: Methods and Critical Appraisal for Evidence-Based Practice*, 9th edition. St Louis: Elsevier pp. 281–304.

An example of using the DJES answers to create an analytical appraisal point

[DESCRIBE] The researchers used a descriptive analysis, using aggregate median scores, inter-quartile ranges, and percentages to describe the results. [JUSTIFY] The median value is commonly chosen for rank data because the mean average is not always appropriate (Sullivan and Artino 2013). [DESCRIBE] The main study results were that research success at an individual level was perceived as adequate (median = 4; IQR 2–6), as was that of the organisation (median = 4; IQR 2–7). However, research success as a team was perceived as less than adequate (median score 2; IQR 1–5). Key barriers to research included 'other work roles take priority' (83%) and 'lack of time for research' (80%), whereas motivators included 'to develop skills' (80%) and 'increased job satisfaction' (63%). [JUSTIFY] Inter-quartile ranges are useful to show the variability of responses around the median value, whereas percentages are a good way to show how many people responded in the same way. [EVALUATE] Descriptive statistics are an excellent way to describe and summarise the data (Sullivan-Bolyai and Bova 2018). Given that the aim of the study was to understand perceptions of research, this approach to analysis seems appropriate. However, it may have been possible to identify and test hypotheses using inferential statistics to make predictions beyond the immediate study data (Sullivan-Bolyai and Bova 2018). This may have improved the generalisability of the findings.

9.6   APPRAISAL OUTCOME

Now that you have worked through the key elements of the study and read around the characteristics of good-quality research, you should be feeling more confident about the study itself, as well as the factors that might have strengthened or limited it. So what next?

If you think back to Chapter 1, research appraisal is not an end point or an activity that happens in isolation. Instead, it is one step in the EBP cycle (see Chapter 2) and its explicit purpose is to determine the relevance or weight that should be given to a piece of evidence. Your appraisal work therefore should lead you to a conclusion on the quality of the study overall. We discussed in earlier chapters how challenging it can feel to critique a published piece of research, but the DJES too can help you here again.

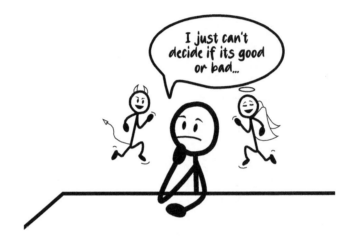

Once you've covered all the elements, look back across all the appraisal points you constructed using the DJES tool. Consider how many points are broadly positive and how many are negative. Have you mainly pointed out limitations of the study? Or have you predominantly highlighted robust method choices and a well-conducted design? Looking across your points can help you then to conclude:

- That the study quality is overall good, perhaps with some minor limitations.
- That the study is significantly limited, although it perhaps tackles an important topic, offers a starting point for other research, or generates some useful findings.
- That the study is mixed, with elements of both.

It's a good idea to include this appraisal outcome in your assignment, as it will further demonstrate that you have developed critical research appraisal skills and can practically apply them to a study.

Remember that the assignment advice given in this text is based on the general requirements of appraisal assignments at academic level 5. In terms of your own assignment, it's important to follow your specific assessment brief and to clarify with your module tutors if there are any other requirements that you should be working towards. For example, do you need to provide an initial descriptive overview of the study, or can you just outline it as you work through the appraisal? Are there any particular research elements or quality markers that should be focused on, or can you select what is pertinent to your study? Most assignments will require some connection with current practice, but this could be done within the appraisal or as a separate discussion. We cover application to practice in Chapter 10, but do find out how your tutor expects you to present this.

9.7 END-OF-CHAPTER CHECKPOINT

		Comment/notes
I can identify descriptive-style writing that says what has happened in the study, what has been reported, or other factual statements	Yes/no	
I can identify analytical-style writing that discusses in more depth how or why the issue being identified is important to raise, and provides some interpretation, justification, or judgement	Yes/no	
I understand that appraising a primary study must have some analysis of, for example, the strengths and limitations of the study elements and how they affect the research quality or results	Yes/no	
I understand how using the tool to break down my writing into descriptive and analytical components will help me improve my writing at academic level 5	Yes/no	
I have arrived at a conclusion about the quality of my study, based on my appraisal	Yes/no	
Now look at the assignment brief or discuss with a module leader and determine which of the following key points should be included in your assignment		
An initial descriptive overview of the study	Yes/no	
Appraising all steps of the research process (or just some)	Yes/no	
Key quality markers	Yes/no	

	Comment/notes
Connection with practice, within the appraisal or separately	Yes/no	
Any texts/articles that are considered essential	Yes/no	

On a scale of 1–5, how confident do you feel about the content in this chapter?

9.8   CHAPTER SUMMARY

This chapter has helped you to develop a better understanding of academic level 5 expectations and the difference between descriptive and analytical writing. You should now be aware that both writing styles are essential, but that your level 5 work needs also to demonstrate your ability to critically evaluate information, to provide informed interpretation of it, and to apply it to a professional context. You've also been provided with a tool to help you construct analytical appraisal points for your assignment and to reach a conclusion on its quality. Now use the end-of-chapter checkpoint to ensure you are feeling confident to begin writing about the appraisal of your own study, and then get going!

REFERENCES

Backmann, M. (2017). What's in a gold standard? In defence of randomised controlled trials. *Medicine, Health Care, and Philosophy* 20: 513–523.

Barrett, D., and Noble, H. (2019). What are cohort studies? *Evidence-Based Nursing* 22 (4): 95–96.

Bedston, S., Akbari, A., Jarvis, C.I. et al. (2022). COVID-19 vaccine uptake, effectiveness, and waning in 82,959 health care workers: a national prospective cohort study in Wales. *Vaccine* 40 (8): 1180–1189.

Comer, C., Collings, R., McCracken, A. et al. (2022). Allied health professionals' perceptions of research in the United Kingdom national health service: a survey of research capacity and culture. *BMC Health Services Research* 22: 1094. https://doi.org/10.1186/s12913-022-08465-6.

Doyle, L., McCabe, C., Keogh, B. et al. (2020). An overview of the qualitative descriptive design within nursing research. *Journal of Research in Nursing* 25 (5): 443–455.

Ferrarello, F., Viligiardi, M., and Di Bari, M. (2018). Ethics reporting practices in randomized controlled trials of physical therapy interventions after stroke. *Archives of Physiotherapy* 8: 1–10.

Flood, A. (2010) Understanding phenomenology. *Nurse Researcher* 17 (2): 7–15.

Goodman, C. and Evans, C. (2015). Focus groups. In: *The Research Process in Nursing*, 7e (ed. K. Gerrish and J. Lathleen), 401–412. Chichester: Wiley Blackwell.

Heale, R., and Forbes, D. (2013). Understanding triangulation in research. *Evidence-Based Nursing* 16 (4): 98–99.

Jones, M. and Rattray, J. (2015). Questionnaire design. In: *The Research Process in Nursing*, 7e (ed. K. Gerrish and J. Lathleen), 413–426. Chichester: Wiley Blackwell.

Mills, E.J., Ayers, D., Chou, R., and Thorlund, K. (2015). Are current standards of reporting quality for clinical trials sufficient in addressing important sources of bias? *Contemporary Clinical Trials* 45: 2–7.

Morse, J.M. (2000, 2000). Determining sample size. *Qualitative Health Research* 10 (1): 3–5.

Newton, K., Dumville, J., Briggs, M. et al. (2022). Postoperative packing of perianal abscess cavities (PPAC2): randomized clinical trial. *British Journal of Surgery* 109 (10): 951–957.

Nursing & Midwifery Council (NMC). (2018). The Code: professional standards of practice and behaviour for nurses, midwives and nursing associates. `https://www.nmc.org.uk/standards/code` (accessed 4 December 2023).

Polit, D. and Beck, C.T. (2021). *Nursing Research: Generating and Assessing Evidence for Nursing Practice*, 11e. Philadelphia: Wolters Kluwer.

Pryce-Miller, M., Bliss, E., Airey, A. et al. (2023). The lived experiences of racial bias for black, Asian and minority ethnic students in practice: a hermeneutic phenomenological study. *Nurse Education in Practice* 66: 103532.

Quality Assurance Agency for Higher Education (2014). *The Frameworks for HE Qualifications of UK Degree-Awarding Bodies*. London: QAA.

Setia, M.S. (2016). Methodology series module 1: cohort studies. *Indian Journal of Dermatology* 61 (1): 21–25.

Shimp, K.M. (2017). Systematic review of turnover/retention and staff perception of staffing and resource adequacy related to staffing. *Nursing Economics* 35 (5): 239–258.

Sullivan, G.M. and Artino, A.R. (2013). Analyzing and interpreting data from Likert-type scales. *Journal of Graduate Medical Education* 5 (4): 541–542. `https://doi.org/10.4300/JGME-5-4-18`.

Sullivan-Bolyai, S. and Bova, C. (2018). Data analysis: descriptive and inferential statistics. In: LoBiondo-Wood, G. and Haber, J. (eds.) *Nursing Research: Methods and Critical Appraisal for Evidence-Based Practice*, 9th edition. St Louis: Elsevier pp. 281–304

Teherani, A., Martimianakis, T., Stenfors-Hayes, T. et al. (2015). Choosing a qualitative research approach. *Journal of Graduate Medical Education* (4): 669–670.

Tipton, E., Hallberg, K., Hedges, L.V., and Chan, W. (2016, 2017). Implications of small samples for generalization: adjustments and rules of thumb. *Evaluation Review* 41 (5): 472–505.

Zemlak, J.L., Alexander, K.A., Wilson, D., and Sherman, S.G. (2023). Contraceptive decision-making through the lens of social determinants of health among female sex workers: a qualitative descriptive study. *Journal of Advanced Nursing* 79: 1898–1911.

CHAPTER 10

Appraisal in Context

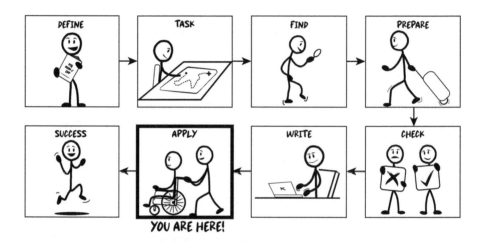

FIVE THINGS TO LEARN FROM THIS CHAPTER

1. Primary research is just one piece in the EBP jigsaw and a single study is rarely sufficient evidence on its own for influencing practice.

2. Evidence synthesis is a collection of multiple pieces of evidence, which have been appraised and analysed to give a conclusion on a particular topic. Secondary research such as systematic reviews and guidelines are examples.

Critical Appraisal Skills for Healthcare Students: A Practical Guide to Writing Evidence-based Practice Assignments, First Edition. Charlotte J. Whiffin, Donna Barnes, and Lorraine Henshaw.
© 2024 John Wiley & Sons Ltd. Published 2024 by John Wiley & Sons Ltd.

3. Evidence implementation is a complex, long-term process of putting the knowledge from evidence into practice to inform care or service delivery.
4. Barriers to evidence implementation include inaccessible research, lack of protected time for healthcare teams to discuss how evidence applies to their setting, and ineffective organisational change processes.
5. Despite the barriers, using evidence to inform, challenge, and advance practice is a powerful tool in healthcare that enables practitioners to be agents of change, improve practice, and be the leaders of tomorrow.

FIVE MINUTES WITH ABIGAIL, OPERATING DEPARTMENT PRACTICE STUDENT

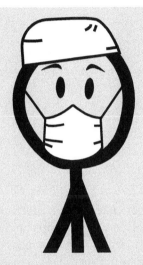

How has learning about appraisal and research been relevant to your development as a registered practitioner?
My research assignments were my favourite assignments. I even recently applied for a job in research! I like that you get to consider a range of evidence on one issue, you can weigh it all up together and make a decision overall.

Do you see change in practice as a result of research?
I sometimes ask why something in practice is done in a particular way as evidence suggests another way. Sometimes the response is 'that's how we have always done it'. I find some staff don't engage in evidence regularly and follow outdated guidance.

Recently we had evidence-based quality improvements where we all now have different-coloured hats in theatre as per our role, these include our name and role. They came from the human factors initiative to improve communication.

What do you think the barriers to health professionals using evidence are?

Cost is also a big barrier but also time too. You don't even tend to see journals in clinical staff rooms or rest areas any more for people to leaf through. These informal ways of connecting with evidence are helpful. I think if there was a link person who could explain and focus all the evidence on a topic that would be helpful too.

There is also a feeling of lacking the influence to create change. Most decisions are made centrally within the organisation and converted into organisational and local policies.

In what assignment did you have to write about EBP?

For the EBP module. Title of assignment was: Critique a suitable article relating to evidence-based practice in health and/or social care and discuss its application to perioperative care.

What advice would you give to students learning about EBP for the first time?

Try to not get overwhelmed, it will all make sense in the end. If you are unsure of anything, ask your module tutor.

10.1   INTRODUCTION

This chapter brings us full circle back to our starting point of EBP. We began by exploring what evidence is and why it's important. We then moved on to primary research evidence specifically, examining the characteristics of qualitative and quantitative methodologies and outlining the main research designs in the 'Key Facts' sections. Zoning in on research appraisal, we used the EDECA model to focus on issues of quality, applicability, and ethical integrity. We then provided the DJES tool and some examples to help you work through your studies and construct your own appraisal points.

So are we nearly there yet? Well, the end is in sight, but we haven't quite arrived!

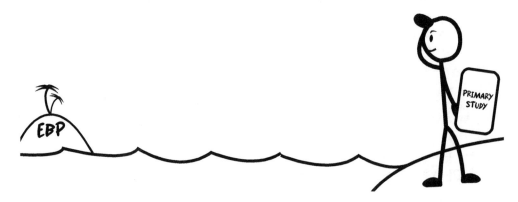

Now we need to consider how to connect the primary research study you've appraised with the real-world practice context. Practical use of research evidence is, after all, the end goal of appraisal. This chapter discusses the 'bridge' or connection between primary research and practice by explaining two key concepts: **evidence synthesis** and **evidence implementation**.

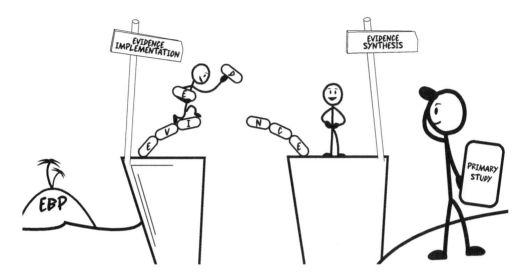

As we think about applying evidence to practice, we are brought back to the starting point of EBP. In Chapter 2, we discussed how EBP was defined as the *conscientious* use of evidence (Sackett et al. 1996). This conscientiousness means that for EBP to be safe and effective, research should not just be appraised and applied. It must also be considered alongside relevant clinical expertise, patient preference, and other factors specific to the care context (Mackey and Bassendowski 2017), which include the local processes, resources, and the wider principles of ethics and law (see the advanced model of EBP in Chapter 2).

Contextual factors such as resources and organisational processes can sometimes inhibit the implementation of evidence in practice, and towards the end of this chapter we explore both barriers to implementation and ways of addressing them. The chapter ends by encouraging you to consider how you might discuss the practice implications of your study appraisal and implementation issues in your assignment.

10.2   THE RELATIONSHIP BETWEEN PRIMARY RESEARCH AND EBP

We've explained that research appraisal is just one step in the EBP cycle and that it has a specific role, which is to determine the relevance or weight that should be given to a piece of research evidence *within a broader evidence base* (Aveyard and Sharp 2017). There are few historical examples of single studies that have produced overwhelming evidence to the extent that they could lead to practice change (Dodgson 2017). Even if their quality is excellent, single studies are generally not powerful or comprehensive enough to generate results with sufficient certainty that they could be applied without considering what other evidence suggests. Most studies are limited in some way and tend to investigate only one population or setting, therefore taken in isolation the findings could be misleading.

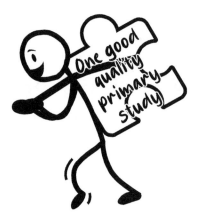

It is more appropriate to think of primary studies as pieces of a jigsaw, each contributing to, and expanding on, the wider evidence base on a topic. The more research that is conducted, the more we see the 'big picture'. This might be that there is a 'consensus' or agreement of findings across many studies. Or the overall evidence base may show a range of different or opposing findings. In this case, the big picture is telling us that we should be cautious about implementing them in practice.

So if EBP requires a collection of research on a topic, how do busy healthcare professionals go about gathering, appraising, and interpreting it all? This is where 'evidence synthesis' comes in.

 Assignment Tip

It is often useful to reflect on the difficulties of implementing research into practice and how likely it is that the study you appraised will influence change. For ideas on this, make sure you read the 'discussion' section of the study. In this part, the researchers should suggest how their findings fit with the current evidence base and practice, and they may reference helpful sources related to the topic for you to look up and explore.

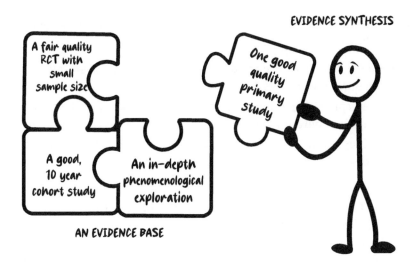

AN EVIDENCE BASE

10.3   EVIDENCE SYNTHESIS

Evidence synthesis can be considered an umbrella term that includes a range of different types of secondary research or literature reviews. In Chapter 2 we introduced you to the Cochrane Collaboration and the importance of systematic reviews to EBP. Look back at Chapter 2 if you need a quick refresher.

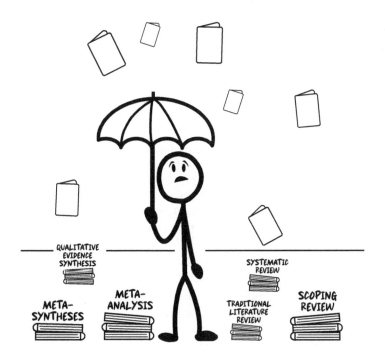

These different types of secondary research typically incorporate all or some of the following characteristics:

- A methodical and transparent search for relevant evidence to answer a focused research question (like we described in Chapter 3).
- A synthesis process that includes appraising the quality of the evidence, before extracting and analysing the findings.
- A goal of providing a reliable summary of relevant evidence that identifies consensus, disagreement, and any gaps – that is, what is not yet known about the issue (Florczak 2018).

The field of evidence synthesis continues to evolve, with new types being used across different disciplines regularly (Munn et al. 2023). Sutton et al. (2019) found 48 distinct types of evidence syntheses, the most commonly used being traditional or generic literature reviews, systematic reviews, and qualitative meta-syntheses. The main differences between these often lies in how systematically the search is conducted, how comprehensive the included evidence is, whether critical appraisal is completed, and how objective the overall process is (Littell 2018). See Table 10.1 for more details.

TABLE 10.1   Common types of review designs.

Type of review	
Traditional reviews or generic literature reviews	A methodical collection and analysis of different types of published research and other literature. Wide variation in degree of comprehensiveness.
Systematic reviews with/ without meta-analysis	An appraisal and synthesis of quantitative research evidence, typically gathered by following an established and rigorous review methodology that aims to reduce bias and increase reliability to answer a focused question relating to the evidence base on the topic. A meta-analysis may or may not be included – this involves the statistical reanalysis of the selected research data, to generate more powerful and precise results.
Qualitative evidence synthesis, or meta-syntheses	An appraisal and synthesis of qualitative research evidence, typically gathered by following an established and rigorous review methodology. This may be a purposeful methodology and the overarching aim is to integrate the research findings to answer a focused question relating to the evidence base on the topic. A meta-synthesis goes one step further and aims to generate new knowledge from the qualitative evidence base.
Scoping review	A review that aims to locate and characterise the evidence base, mapping out its key features and identifying areas for more research.
Integrative literature reviews	Allows the combination of different research methodologies e.g. qualitative and quantitative. Useful where the review question is broad and the evidence base is mixed.

Regardless of the type, good-quality syntheses play a crucial role in supporting health professionals' use of evidence as well as being invaluable sources for informing future research, service delivery, and policy. These need to be appraised just like primary research.

 Explore It!

You can find appraisal tools for reviews in the same place as tools to critique primary research. Check out the tools from the Critical Skills Appraisal Programme, the Joanna Briggs Institute, and the Centre for Evidence-Based Medicine:

```
https://casp-uk.net/casp-tools-checklists
https://jbi.global/critical-appraisal-tools
https://www.cebm.ox.ac.uk/resources/ebm-tools/
critical-appraisal-tools
```

 Assignment Tip

Any type of literature review is a useful source of evidence. Use these in all your assignments and make a point of telling the marker that you have used a literature review and what type of review this is. If it is a Cochrane review, be sure to point this out too. For example:

In a systematic review by Ali et al. (2023) artificial intelligence was found to be more accurate than human performance.

In a Cochrane review and meta-analysis to evaluate the effects of interventions to prevent the use of physical restraints, organisational interventions were likely to reduce the use of physical restraints (Möhler et al. 2023).

Evidence syntheses also contribute to clinical guidelines. Clinical guidelines are systematically developed recommendations for patient care that present management strategies relating to a particular condition (Thomas 1999). They can be locally or nationally produced guidelines such as those developed by the National Institute for Health and Care Excellence (NICE) and the Scottish Intercollegiate Guidelines Network (SIGN), and they typically use independent committees to conduct a rigorous process of gathering, appraising, and synthesising evidence. The committees comprise a range of people and organisations related to the guideline topic to ensure that as many perspectives as possible are considered. They typically include health professionals, academics, care providers, and commissioners, as well as those using health services and their family members or carers (NICE 2023; SIGN 2021).

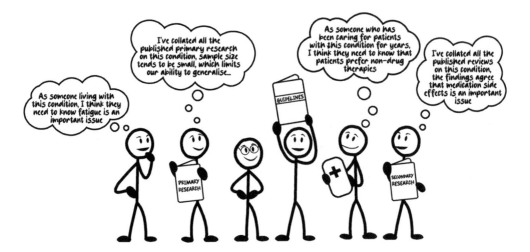

As well as providing a digestible set of evidence-based recommendations, assessed by key stakeholders, guidelines are also developed with implementation in mind (Beauchemin et al. 2019). While research is commonly criticised for lacking clinical relevance or usefulness (Gerrish 2015; Ioannidis 2016), guidelines explicitly aim to provide practical recommendations for those delivering care.

 Explore It!

Visit the NICE or SIGN website to read more about how clinical guidelines are developed using the best available research:

www.nice.org.uk/about/what-we-do/our-programmes/nice-guidance/nice-guidelines/how-we-develop-nice-guidelines

www.sign.ac.uk/what-we-do/methodology/new-developments

As with all types of evidence, guidelines need to be appraised by the clinicians using them in terms of their suitability to the setting they are being used in. Despite being rigorously developed and a credible synthesis of information, guidelines are by no means 'perfect'. Evidence may be outdated by the point of implementation, the guidelines may be unsuitable for the patient group, or they may not be feasible in terms of cost or time for some settings to implement (Johansson et al. 2023). These criticisms do not detract from the value of guidelines for EBP. Instead, the points emphasise the central principle of EBP, that all evidence must be carefully considered in terms of quality and applicability before being implemented.

Explore It!

As with all forms of evidence, there is a tool to help appraise guidelines, 'Appraisal of Guidelines, Research and Evaluation' (AGREE). The first version was released in 2003 and this was later updated by Brouwers et al. (2010) to AGREE II.

You can access the AGREE II tool, and additional resources, on the AGREE website: `https://www.agreetrust.org/agree-ii`

10.4   EVIDENCE IMPLEMENTATION

10.4.1   Translating Evidence into Practice

Having retrieved and appraised the evidence, the next step is to translate the findings into practice so that patients, professionals, and healthcare services benefit from this new knowledge. You may think this next step is straightforward, but we have a few more challenges to overcome before we reach our end goal.

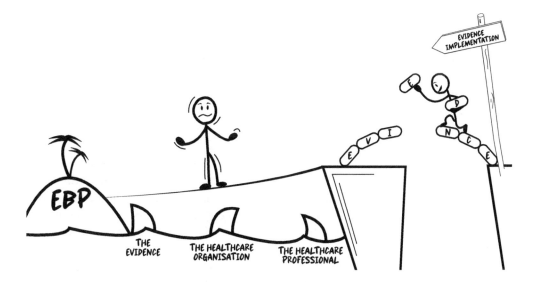

It is well recognised, nationally and internationally, that implementing evidence in healthcare settings is difficult (Curtis et al. 2017). It is a complex, long-term process that requires the active participation of many different members of a healthcare organisation, while these professionals continue with their everyday work and manage the fluctuating pressures of contemporary healthcare. In fact, the field of 'implementation science' has emerged to investigate the barriers that make the use of evidence so challenging and to find practical solutions to address them (Theobald et al. 2018). Haines et al. (2004) have described how barriers to EBP can happen at any point in the journey, from the development of the research to the point at which it meets the health professionals and patients in the clinical setting. Think about factors that could be preventing the implementation of evidence as you work through the next Checkpoint Activity.

 Aim: To examine the factors that make implementing evidence in practice challenging

Instructions: Read the case study and make notes on the possible barriers to implementing the evidence.

Case study: Evidence on pre-operative fasting times in the UK

Hewson and Moppett (2020) are both anaesthetists working in Nottingham in the East Midlands who have written about the issue of pre-operative fasting times. They have explored how fasting before a surgical operation developed as an effective way of reducing the risk of pulmonary aspiration (inhalation of fluid or particles into the lungs). The general anaesthetic given before surgery inhibits the reflex action of the larynx and can lead to regurgitation of the stomach contents. If this happens during surgery, it can be fatal or can lead to serious complications, such as infection and respiratory fibrosis.

Initially, making a patient 'nil by mouth from midnight' prior to the surgery was seen as the safest way of reducing stomach contents and therefore the risk of pulmonary aspiration. But this ambiguous strategy could be inconsistently applied and could lead to extensive periods without food or fluids when, for example, surgery times were altered (Hewson and Moppett 2020). It was later discovered that although the risk of pulmonary aspiration was reduced, prolonged fasting could result in patient harm from dehydration and electrolyte imbalance, hypoglycaemia, and impaired post-operative recovery (Liddle 2014).

Such adverse outcomes prompted many primary studies to investigate the safest, shortest fasting time, and over the past 30 years the evidence base on this has grown. Now there is agreement across international evidence syntheses that fasting patients from midnight the night before surgery is unnecessary. A systematic review (Brady et al. 2003) and clinical guidelines from the European Society of Anaesthesiology (Smith et al. 2011) and the American Society of Anaesthesiologists (2017) all suggest that adult patients should eat food no closer than six hours before anaesthesia and they should be encouraged to drink appropriate fluids until two hours before anaesthesia (Hewson and Moppett 2020). Despite this high-quality evidence consensus and an apparent lack of opposition to the recommendations, audits show that fasting is still occurring for much longer durations (Hewson and Moppett 2020).

Barriers to EBP: What factors can you think of that may explain why this evidence has not been implemented in practice? Make your notes and then read on to find out more about what inhibits research implementation and what can facilitate it.

10.4.2   Barriers to Implementing Evidence

The Hewson and Moppett (2020) case study is interesting because it seems to have all the 'ingredients' for successful EBP and yet the evidence has not quite made it across the final hurdle into practice. This suggests that there are other barriers that are preventing implementation. The barriers can be categorised in terms of factors relating to the evidence itself, factors relating to the organisational context, and factors relating to the individual healthcare professional (McNett et al. 2022; Naghibi et al. 2021; Gerrish 2015; Haines et al. 2004). Let's consider these now alongside some strategies to address them.

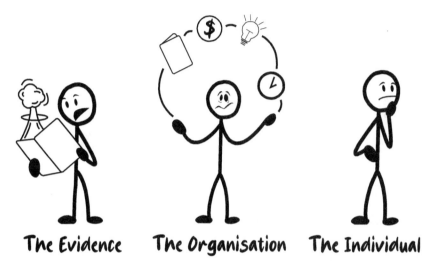

The Evidence   The Organisation   The Individual

10.4.2.1   Implementation Barrier: The Evidence

Research has been criticised for being too disconnected from real-world healthcare settings and for not making the practice implications clear enough (Marshall 2014). Evidence syntheses and clinical guidelines partly address this problem by gathering and appraising large volumes of research and isolating the implications for practice. Another way of making research more relevant is to encourage and support health professionals to undertake research themselves (Marshall 2014). This makes it more likely that pertinent clinical issues are researched in the first place, and that a study report will clearly highlight the practical implications of the findings.

The fact that research is generally communicated though academic journals and conferences also creates a barrier, as most health professionals infrequently read or attend them (Titler 2008; Gerrish 2015). However, rapid developments in technology-mediated communication are already challenging these traditions. Researchers, health professionals, and academics have made good use of social media, disseminating evidence more widely, quickly, and in more accessible formats than ever before. Blogs, podcasts, mini-films, and visual abstracts are now often used to provide an overview of research in an accessible and visually appealing way and to encourage engagement and discussion about the findings (Ramos and Concepcion 2020).

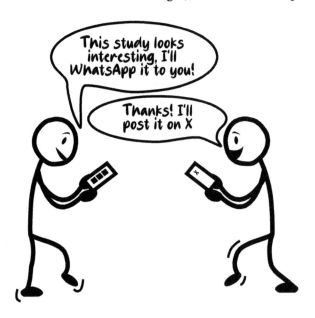

 Explore It!

Check out these examples of visual abstracts from the Centers for Disease Control and Prevention (CDC):

> https://www.cdc.gov/genomics/visual/visual_abstract.htm

10.4.2.2   Implementation Barrier: The Organisation

Organisational processes and cultures significantly influence the implementation of evidence. In today's high-pressure clinical environments, there is limited space and time to gather, appraise, and discuss evidence, and to consider as a team how it might be applied. Furthermore, organisational cultures can inhibit EBP changes. Hierarchical organisational structures take a 'top-down' approach to change, meaning that it tends to be driven by senior leaders rather than front-line staff. Such processes are less effective for EBP because front-line staff are distanced from the rationale and evidence underpinning the change (Gallagher-Ford 2014).

Organisational culture shifts are notoriously challenging, but there is increasing acknowledgement and support for front-line staff to make evidence-based changes. For example, there are several frameworks that have been developed to support organisations with facilitating EBP. The Promoting Action on Research Implementation in Health Services (PARIHS) framework (Kitson et al. 2008), the Consolidated

Framework for Implementation Research model (Damschroder et al. 2009), and the Knowledge to Action framework (Graham and Tetroe 2010) are just a few examples.

Providing healthcare professionals with access to EBP resources is a key part of facilitating the use of evidence within organisations. These include health librarians, relevant training, software, and, perhaps most importantly, protected time as a health-care team to discuss evidence in relation to local needs. Running journal clubs is one way of providing this protected time. These have been trialled by several UK NHS Trusts and evidence is growing in terms of their effectiveness for supporting EBP (Kjerholt and Hølge-Hazelton 2018).

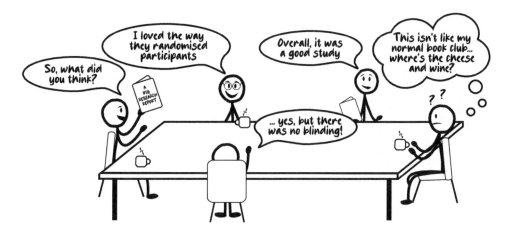

 Assignment Tip

Consider including some reflection on the organisational cultures you have been exposed to in practice, for example whether they promote EBP and what strategies they use. Make your writing more analytical by supporting and expanding your points using texts and articles that discuss theories of EBP cultures within healthcare organisations.

10.4.2.3   Implementation Barrier: Healthcare Professionals

Lastly, it is important to consider the contribution of healthcare professionals themselves – in other words, you! Individuals may feel they lack EBP skills or may have some anxieties or negative perceptions about research. 'Resistance to change' is often cited as a barrier to health professionals implementing evidence, but what does this mean? An individual's ability to manage change may be influenced by personal values or their previous experiences of change. They might also feel that the suggested change implies their previous practice was wrong, making them feel criticised.

It's important therefore to explore our own feelings about using evidence. Reflection has been suggested as one way of doing this, as it is a process of making sense of, and learning from, our own clinical experiences (Thompson and Burns 2008).

Healthcare professionals might use a recent scenario where they were unsure how to manage a patient situation, or where they were unclear about a plan of care or treatment. Making time to think through the issues, bringing in related research and evidence, can encourage future use of evidence in practice.

While it's crucial for individuals to examine their attitudes to EBP and identify areas to strengthen, implementing research in practice is ultimately a team effort. Even where individuals have advanced research skills, providing evidence-based health services requires all health professionals to take an active role. Working collaboratively as a team can impact on the quality of care for all patients, but it can also be the most effective strategy for EBP. Within a team, members will have a range of skills, experience, and knowledge, and pooling these collectively can strengthen individual efforts.

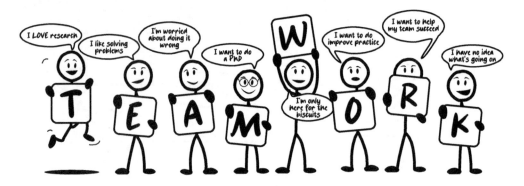

10.5   WRITING ABOUT EVIDENCE IMPLEMENTATION IN YOUR ASSIGNMENT

While you should check the requirements for your assignments, most appraisal assessments will expect some discussion about evidence implementation, or the relationship between evidence and healthcare practice more generally. This is because the practical use of research evidence in health settings is the end goal of research appraisal and the EBP process. A discussion of evidence implementation can take many forms, as long as you demonstrate understanding of the key principles set out in this chapter and that even with a good range of quality evidence, ensuring that practice is actually informed by it are needed. We will give you two suggestions for how you might present such evidence here.

First, you could keep your discussion specific to the research you have appraised, considering the primary study findings (or one aspect of them) in relation to the broader evidence base. For example, you might conduct a basic search for secondary research, perhaps a systematic review or meta-synthesis on your topic, and some guidelines or local polices. You could then use these to support a discussion about how your wider evidence aligns with, or contradicts, the findings of the primary study. If you have a topic where there is little other evidence, perhaps because it is an emerging issue, then make this your discussion point. Explain why a lack of evidence is problematic for health professionals. See the examples that follow for how some students have done this.

Second, you could present a more general discussion of the principles of evidence implementation. This is more likely to require supporting sources in the form of textbooks and journal articles, and may not involve any additional research evidence or further discussion of the primary research you appraised. It may instead include a broader discussion of EBP, such as the professional requirement, the importance of evidence synthesis, the barriers to implementation, and a reflection on your own professional practice or what you have seen in healthcare settings.

10.6   ASSIGNMENT EXAMPLES

Example 1: Although this was one primary study, Mitchell et al.'s (2021) findings are reflected in other evidence, including a systematic review (Malcolm et al. 2020). A systematic review is a stronger form of evidence, which gathers and synthesises multiple studies on a particular topic (Clarke 2011). Malcolm et al. (2020) found that while there is a growing international trend to bring children's palliative care treatments closer to their homes, parents needed improved access to specialised palliative care experts to enable them to remain in their roles as parents, and to be given the option of receiving end-of-life care at home (Malcolm et al. 2020). However, more research is still needed to improve paediatric palliative care in practice (Mitchell et al. 2021). The National Institute for Health and Care Excellence (2016) guidelines also call for more research to inform both practice and policy development so that palliative care of children at home and in hospital can be updated and improved (Mitchell et al. 2021; NICE 2016).

Example 2: Sharma et al.'s (2021) findings were supported by another primary study (Ceyar et al. 2020), also with a small sample size, which found that knotless barbed sutures reduced suturing time, facilitated wound closure and minimised complications. However, the National Institute for Health and Care Excellence (NICE) issued guidance in 2021 which concluded that that evidence base was very mixed and was dependent on the type of surgery and the outcome measured by the study (NICE 2021). This guidance was based on 31 randomised controlled trials and therefore offered stronger evidence on the issue. The lack of definitive findings makes clinical decision-making on suture type difficult. When discussing this issue in practice, I found that the surgical team were aware of the research evidence but they also had different perspectives, based on their clinical experience. They were concerned about cost implications and possible additional workload if removal of barbed sutures was required. Therefore, to improve EBP on the issue of suture type, more research needs to be undertaken with larger sample sizes and it should investigate the issues that concern the healthcare professionals in this field.

Example 3: Squires et al. (2019) suggests that certain barriers exist, with access to EBP resources and lack of time being identified as the most common. Fitzpatrick (2007) argues that organisations must enable the development of EBP within the workplace and facilitate team collaboration to improve evidence-based decision-making and enhance the delivery of care (Athanasakis 2013).

Example 4: Integrating research into healthcare practice has many advantages (Ellis 2011), including improved patient outcomes and increased professional accountability, and providing HCPs with evidence-based rationale on which to inform clinical decisions. However, a range of barriers, including a lack of organisational support and time constraints, can impede the successful utilisation of research findings (Kerr and Rainey 2021). My practice setting has a strong EBP culture which actively encourages the dissemination of best practice guidance and updated research findings through regular team meetings and evidence champions. This type of organisational support is crucial to facilitate EBP and promote a culture of seeking, sharing and using quality evidence for practice (Hood 2018).

10.7   END-OF-CHAPTER CHECKPOINT

		Comment/notes
I can discuss the limitations of primary research for informing practice	Yes/No	
I can describe the principles of evidence synthesis and why a range of evidence is important for informing practice	Yes/No	
I can identify some barriers to evidence implementation	Yes/No	
I can suggest some strategies that may improve evidence implementation	Yes/No	
I have checked in the assignment brief/with my module leader if a broader discussion of evidence implementation is expected in my assignment, and if so how much	Yes/No	
If the answer to the above is YES		
I have checked in the assignment brief/with my module leader if the discussion of evidence implementation should be applied to my appraised study topic, or if it should be more general	Yes/No	
On a scale of 1–5 how confident do you feel the content in this chapter?		

10.8   YOU MADE IT TO THE END. . . OR IS IT?

Congratulations, you've made it to the end of your EBP journey! You've understood the concept of EBP, acquired some research evidence, gathered your supportive tools, evaluated its quality, and written up the appraisal before finally considering how that relates to the real world of healthcare practice. Well done!

You now have everything you need to write a great EBP assignment and the foundation to understand and use evidence in professional practice. This may be the end of this journey for now, but it is not the end of EBP as you move to higher academic levels and continue your journey as a registered professional.

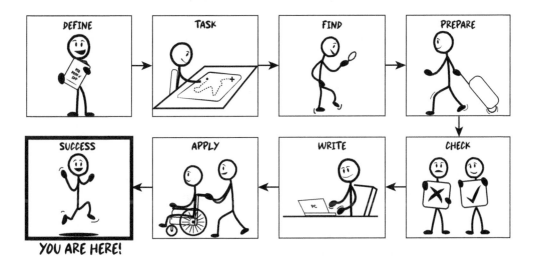

10.9   FINAL WORDS OF WISDOM

Despite the barriers, using evidence to inform, challenge, and advance practice is a powerful tool in healthcare that enables practitioners to be agents of change, improve practice, and be the leaders of tomorrow. We hope that our passion, enthusiasm, and experience support you to get the best out of this learning experience and that you take a love for research with you through your professional life. We hope that this book is just the beginning, and that we have given you both the knowledge and the confidence to explore some of the more advanced research concepts that underpin the generation of new knowledge. But be warned, this can be like opening Pandora's box that reveals more complex and complicated research theory! Don't forget that you can immerse yourself fully and unapologetically in all its wonder or be pragmatic and stay in the shallow end. The choice is yours.

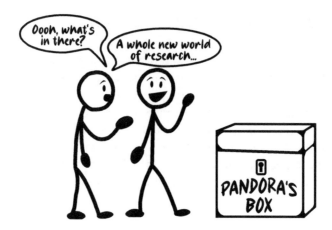

If you still don't believe in the power of EBP and critical appraisal, here is a final word from one of our students:

Keep an open mind and keep positive. Put in the work and you will achieve a good outcome.

REFERENCES

Ali, O., Abdelbaki, W., Shrestha, A. et al. (2023). A systematic literature review of artificial intelligence in the healthcare sector: benefits, challenges, methodologies, and functionalities. *Journal of Innovation & Knowledge* 8 (1): 100333.

American Society of Anesthesiologists (2017). Practice guidelines for preoperative fasting and the use of pharmacologic agents to reduce the risk of pulmonary aspiration: application to healthy patients undergoing elective procedures. *Anesthesiology* 126: 376–393.

Athanasakis, E. (2013). Nurses' research behaviour and barriers to research utilisation into clinical nursing practice: a closer look. *International Journal of Caring Sciences* 6 (1): 16–28.

Aveyard, H. and Sharp, P. (2017). *A Beginner's Guide to Evidence-Based Practice in Health and Social Care*, 3e. London: Open University Press.

Beauchemin, M., Cohn, E., and Shelton, R.C. (2019). Implementation of clinical practice guidelines in the health care setting: a concept analysis. *ANS Advance Nursing Science* 42 (4): 307–324. https://doi.org/10.1097/ANS.0000000000000263.

Brady, M.C., Kinn, S., Stuart, P., and Ness, V. (2003). Preoperative fasting for adults to prevent perioperative complications. *Cochrane Database Systematic Review* (4): CD004423. https://doi.org/10.1002/14651858.CD004423.

Brouwers, M.C., Kho, M.E., Browman, G.P. et al. (2010). AGREE next steps consortium. AGREE II: advancing guideline development, reporting and evaluation in health care. *CMAJ* 182: E839–E842. https://doi.org/10.1503/cmaj.090449.20603348.

Ceyar, K.R., Thulasidoss, G.P., Cheeman, S.R.S. et al. (2020). Effectiveness of knotless suture as a wound closure agent for impacted third molara split mouth randomized controlled clinical trial. *Journal of Cranio-Maxillofacial Surgery* 48 (10): 1004–1008.

Clarke, J. (2011). What is a systematic review? *Evidence-Based Nursing* 14 (3): 64. https://doi.org/10.1136/ebn.2011.0049.

Curtis, K., Fry, M., Shaban, R.Z., and Considine, J. (2017). Translating research findings to clinical nursing practice. *Journal of Clinical Nursing* 26 (5–6): 862–872.

Damschroder, L.J., Aron, D.C., Keith, R.E. et al. (2009). Fostering implementation of health services research findings into practice: a consolidated framework for advancing implementation science. *Implementation Science* 4 (1): 1–15.

Dodgson, J. (2017). Should one study change practice? *Journal of Human Lactation* 33 (3): 476–477.

Ellis, P. (2011). *Understanding Research for Nursing Students*. Exeter: Learning Matters.

Fitzpatrick, J. (2007). How to turn research into evidence-based practice part three: making a case. *Nursing Times* 103 (19): 32–33. https://www.nursingtimes.net/roles/nurse-managers/how-to-turn-research-into-evidence-based-practice-part-three-making-a-case-09-05-2007.

Florczak, K. (2018). Qualitative synthesis: ontological care please. *Nursing Science Quarterly* 31 (3): 220–223. https://doi.org/10.1177/0894318418774869.

Gallagher-Ford, L. (2014). Implementing and sustaining EBP in real world healthcare settings: a leader's role in creating a strong context for EBP. *Worldviews on Evidence-Based Nursing* 11 (1): 72–74.

Gerrish, K. (2015). Translating research findings into practice. In: *The Research Process in Nursing*, 7e (ed. K. Gerrish and J. Lathlean), 555–570. Chichester: Wiley Blackwell.

Graham, I.D. and Tetroe, J.M. (2010). The knowledge to action framework. In: *Models and Frameworks for Implementing Evidence-Based Practice: Linking Evidence to Action* (ed. J. Rycroft-Malone and T. Bucknall), 207–222. Chichester: Wiley.

Haines, A., Haines, A., and Donald, A. (ed.) (2004). *Getting Research Findings into Practice*. Chichester: Wiley.

Hewson, D.W. and Moppett, I. (2020). Preoperative fasting and prevention of pulmonary aspiration in adults: research feast, quality improvement famine. *British Journal of Anaesthesia* 124 (4): 361–363.

Hood, L. (2018). *Leddy and Pepper's Professional Nursing*, 9e. Philadelphia: Wolters Kluwer.

Ioannidis, J.P.A. (2016). Why most clinical research is not useful. *PLoS Medicine* 13 (6): e1002049. https://doi.org/10.1371/journal.pmed.1002049.

Johansson, M., Guyatt, G., and Montori, V. (2023). Guidelines should consider clinicians' time needed to treat. *British Medical Journal* 380: e072953. https://doi.org/10.1136/bmj-2022-072953.

Kerr, H. and Rainey, D. (2021). Addressing the current challenges of adopting evidence-based practice in nursing. *British Journal of Nursing* 30 (16): 970–974. https://doi.org/10.12968/bjon.2021.30.16.970.

Kitson, A.L., Rycroft-Malone, J., Harvey, G. et al. (2008). Evaluating the successful implementation of evidence into practice using the PARiHS framework: theoretical and practical challenges. *Implementation Science* 3 (1): 7–9.

Kjerholt, M. and Hølge-Hazelton, B. (2018). Cultivating a culture of research in nursing through a journal club for leaders: a pilot study. *Journal of Nursing Management* 26 (1): 42–49.

Liddle, C. (2014). Nil by mouth: best practice and patient education. *Nursing Times* 110 (26): 12–14.

Littell, J.H. (2018). Conceptual and practical classification of research reviews and other evidence synthesis products. *Campbell Systematic Reviews* 14 (1): 1–21. https://doi.org/10.4073/cmdp.2018.1.

Mackey, A. and Bassendowski, S. (2017). The history of evidence-based practice in nursing education and practice. *Journal of Professional Nursing* 33 (1): 51–55.

Malcolm, C., Knighting, K., and Taylor, C. (2020). Home-based end of life care for children and their families – a systematic scoping review and narrative synthesis. *Journal of Pediatric Nursing* 55: 126–133.

Marshall, M. (2014). Bridging the ivory towers and the swampy lowlands; increasing the impact of health services research on quality improvement. *International Journal of Quality in Health Care* 26 (1): 1–5. https://doi.org/10.1093/intqhc/mzt076.

McNett, M., Tucker, S., Zadvinskis, I. et al. (2022). A qualitative force field analysis of facilitators and barriers to evidence-based practice in healthcare using an implementation framework. *Global Implementation Research and Applications* 2 (3): 195–208.

Mitchell, S., Slowther, A., Coad, J. et al. (2021). Facilitators and barriers to the delivery of palliative care to children with life-limiting and life-threatening conditions: a qualitative study of the experiences and perceptions of healthcare professionals. *Archives of Disease in Childhood* 107 (1): 59–64.

Möhler, R., Richter, T., Köpke, S., and Meyer, G. (2023). Interventions for preventing and reducing the use of physical restraints for older people in all long-term care settings. *Cochrane Database of Systematic Reviews* (7): CD007546. https://doi.org/10.1002/14651858.CD007546.pub3.

Munn, Z., Pollock, D., Price, C. et al. (2023). Investigating different typologies for the synthesis of evidence: a scoping review protocol. *JBI Evidence Synthesis* 21 (3): 592–600. https://doi.org/10.11124/JBIES-22-00122.

Naghibi, D., Mohammadzadeh, S., and Azami-Aghdash, S. (2021). Barriers to evidence-based practice in health system: a systematic review. *Evidence Based Care* 11 (2): 74–82.

National Institute for Health and Care Excellence (NICE) (2016). Recommendations: end of life care for infants, children and young people with life-limiting conditions: planning and management: guidance. https://www.nice.org.uk/guidance/ng61/chapter/recommendations (accessed 4 December 2023).

National Institute for Health and Care Excellence (NICE) (2021). NICE recommends adoption of absorbable stitches with antibacterial protection for use on the NHS. https://

www.nice.org.uk/news/nice-medical-technology-guidance-plus-sutures (accessed 4 December 2023).

National Institute for Health and Care Excellence (NICE) (2023). How we develop NICE guidelines. www.nice.org.uk/about/what-we-do/our-programmes/nice-guidance/nice-guidelines/how-we-develop-nice-guidelines (accessed 4 December 2023).

Ramos, E. and Concepcion, P. (2020). Visual abstracts: redesigning the landscape of research dissemination. *Seminars in Nephrology* 40 (3): 291–297.

Sackett, D.L., Rosenberg, W.M.C., Gray, J.A.M. et al. (1996). Evidence based medicine: what it is and what it isn't. *British Medical Journal* 312: 71. https://doi.org/10.1136/bmj.312.7023.71.

Scottish intercollegiate Guidelines Network (SIGN) (2021). What we do. https://www.sign.ac.uk/what-we-do/methodology/new-developments (accessed 4 December 2023).

Sharma, A.K., Doss, G.T., Panneerselvam, E. et al. (2021). Use of knotless barbed sutures for closure of intraoral incisions for maxillofacial trauma: a randomised controlled trial. *British Journal of Oral and Maxillofacial Surgery* 59 (2): e72–e78.

Smith, I., Kranke, P., Murat, I. et al. (2011). Perioperative fasting in adults and children: guidelines from the European Society of Anaesthesiology. *European Journal of Anaesthesiology* 28 (8): 556–569.

Squires, J., Aloisio, L., Grimshaw, J. et al. (2019). Attributes of context relevant to healthcare professionals' use of research evidence in clinical practice: a multi-study analysis. *Implementation Science* 14 (1): 1–14. https://doi.org/10.1186/s13012-019-0900-8.

Sutton, A., Clowes, M., Preston, L., and Booth, A. (2019). Meeting the review family: exploring review types and associated information retrieval requirements. *Health Information and Libraries Journal* 36 (3): 202–222. https://doi.org/10.1111/hir.12276.

Theobald, S., Brandes, N., Gyapong, M. et al. (2018). Implementation research: new imperatives and opportunities in global health. *Lancet* 392 (10160): 2214–2228.

Thomas, L. (1999). Clinical practice guidelines. *Evidence-Based Nursing* 2 (2): 38–39. https://doi.org/10.1136/ebn.2.2.38.

Thompson, D.N. and Burns, H.K. (2008). Reflection: an essential element of evidence-based practice. *Journal of Emergency Nursing* 34 (3): 246–248.

Titler, M.G. (2008). The evidence for evidence-based practice implementation. In: *Patient Safety and Quality: An Evidence-Based Handbook for Nurses* (ed. R.G. Hughes), 497–549. Rockville, MD: Agency for Healthcare Research and Quality.

Appendix

A.1 MIXED METHODS KEY FACTS SHEET

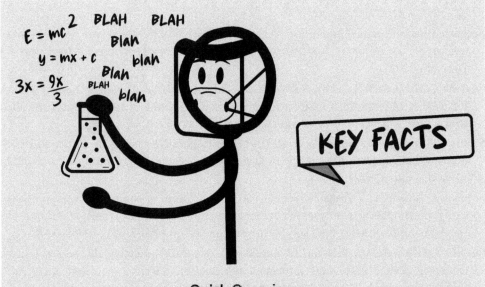

Quick Overview

- Mixed-methods research combines both quantitative and qualitative data collection *and* analysis techniques in one study.
- Mixed-methods research is chosen when generating knowledge from both a quantitative and a qualitative position provides the best, most holistic answer to the research question(s) (Moorley and Cathala 2019).
- Mixed-methods researchers are pragmatic about the different philosophical positions underpinning quantitative and qualitative research and instead concentrate on 'what works' for their research.
- Mixing quantitative and qualitative techniques is not easy and takes skilful consideration of how the different sources of data work together.

- A good mixed-methods study is designed not only to get the best of the two different approaches, optimising the answer to the research question, but also to make the most of the sequencing and integration of data.
- To appraise mixed-methods research, knowledge of quantitative, qualitative, *and* mixed-methods principles and quality markers must be applied.

Aim: To provide a comprehensive understanding of a research topic using a combination of quantitative and qualitative research principles and methods.

Typical research questions/aims: To explore ... *and* measure ...; To examine ... *and* understand ...; To determine the efficacy *and* tolerability of ...

Mixed-methods research questions typically contain both measurable and exploratory components. For example, the question may investigate how participants experienced an intervention as well as how effective it was for reducing symptoms. Efficacy of the intervention for reducing symptoms can be measured (quantitative), but to understand why the intervention may have worked for some and not others requires an exploratory approach (qualitative).

Real Examples

- Predictive factors for depression and anxiety in men during the perinatal period: a mixed methods study (Chhabra et al. 2022).
- Art in occupational therapy education: an exploratory mixed-methods study of an arts-based module (Coppola et al. 2017).
- Premature birth: subjective and psychological experiences in the first weeks following childbirth, a mixed-methods study (Goutaudier et al. 2011).

Three Unique Design Features

1. **Methodological dominance**

   While mixed-methods designs investigate questions that include objective and subjective components and use both qualitative and quantitative methods in one study, these are not always equally balanced. Instead, one methodology may take a primary or secondary role in the study design (Creswell and Plano Clark 2017). The primary or dominant method tends to steer decisions about the research, including what participants to recruit, what data to collect, and how to interpret them.

   An example of a study in which the quantitative method is dominant would be a large, randomised controlled trial with the primary aim of establishing if a new drug causes an effect on arthritis symptoms. However, the secondary study aim is to explore participants' experiences of being in the trial and this requires a qualitative component, such as interviewing a percentage of the participants. This sort of study, where the quantitative methodology is dominant, can be described as 'big QUANT, small qual'. Conversely, a study with the primary aim of interpreting the experience of living with arthritis and a secondary aim of measuring participants' quality of life before and after treatment has qualitative methodology as the dominant approach. It can be described as 'big QUAL, small quant'.

2. **Sequencing**

How the methods are ordered through the research process is also important in understanding a mixed-methods design. A **sequential** mixed-methods design is one that starts and completes one method before beginning another and this is done so that the first method informs the next. For example, a study may first collect data using a focus group method and use the findings to develop questions for a later questionnaire. Similarly, a study may sequence an initial questionnaire and after analysing the data may conduct interviews with participants who had expressed a certain view.

Alternatively, a **concurrent** mixed-methods design means that the quantitative and qualitative methods are conducted at the same time. Often concurrent designs are used when data sets are merged, to provide 'triangulation' or verification of the data. For example, a study measuring physical effects of an intervention by taking blood samples, while exploring the experience of undergoing the intervention using interviews, may conduct both methods at the same time.

3. **Design classifications**

Researchers can choose which methods they use, what weighting they give to each methodology, and how to sequence them, but the overall design will be classified according to four main types. These are embedded, explanatory, exploratory, and triangulation mixed-methods designs (Creswell and Plano Clark 2017).

Embedded designs describe those studies where one methodology is dominant or primary while the other methodology is secondary or plays a more supportive role (for example, a small amount of qualitative data is collected for or embedded within a large randomised controlled trial). The methods can be ordered sequentially or concurrently.

Explanatory designs are always sequential in nature, to connect data from two phases of the study, which tends to be a quantitative phase followed by a qualitative phase.

Exploratory designs are also sequential but tend to begin with a qualitative phase to inform a later quantitative phase.

Lastly, **triangulation** designs are usually concurrent, with the qualitative and quantitative elements contributing equally to answering the research question. The data from both elements are merged during analysis, often revealing points of divergence and convergence (Creswell and Plano Clark 2017) and strengthening the findings overall.

Strengths

Combining both objective and subjective knowledge can facilitate a more holistic or comprehensive answer to a research question if designed well. It is possible to generate and test theories in the same study.

Limitations

Mixed-methods research can be very time-consuming, expensive, and labour intensive. It is often done poorly without proper consideration of how the data sets work together.

EDECA Appraisal Considerations

It is recommended that you appraise each part of the study separately first using the relevant parts of Chapters 7 and 8 for guidance. However, in a similar way to how mixed-methods research integrates qualitative and quantitative elements, you must also combine both aspects of the appraisal into one, so that you can make a judgement on the quality of the study overall.

The following EDECA appraisal considerations review the mixing of methods and how to appraise the approach taken by the researchers.

Ethics

- Was ethical approval/favourable opinion granted for the study?
- Were ethical principles adhered to in terms of consent, confidentiality, and risk versus harm?
- What design decisions were made because of ethical principles?

Design

- Is it clear why a mixed-methods design was used to answer the research question? Hint – look at the question, are there both objective and subjective components?
- Do the authors describe their mixed-methods design (sequential or concurrent? Triangulation, exploratory, explanatory or embedded?) Hint – if it is not explicitly stated, can you tell how the different data components contribute to the study?
- Does one method appear to be more dominant than the other and is this discussed by the authors? Hint – try to a get a feel for which methodological

quality markers are more prevalent in the paper, which will indicate which approach is more dominant.

- Does the study demonstrate both quantitative quality markers of objectivity, validity, reliability, and generalisability *and* qualitative quality markers of subjectivity, credibility, confirmability, and transferability? Go back to Chapters 7 and 8 to review these concepts if you are not confident about what they are.

Enrol

- Are the same participants used for both quantitative and qualitative methods? Hint – in sequential designs the participants may be invited from the same sample as the first phase, but ensure that any overlap is justified.
- Are there enough people in both the qualitative and quantitative approaches to achieve the study aims?
- If the study is trying to generalise from the overall results, do you think the sample is representative?
- If the study is seeking deeper understanding, were the right people invited to participate?

Collect

- How were the data for each method collected and in what order?
- Does the order of data collection reflect the design the authors state that they used?
- Are the quantitative data-collection methods valid and reliable?
- Do the qualitative data-collection methods encourage in-depth and rich responses?

Analyse

- Were appropriate statistical tests used to analyse the quantitative data?
- Did the analysis of the qualitative data deliver an authentic representation of the participants' experiences?
- How were the findings from both data sets used to answer the research question? Hint – did the qualitative findings inform the quantitative data collection (or vice versa) or were the qualitative findings used to confirm the quantitative findings (or vice versa)?
- Are the different data sets consistent, for example did they find similar things, or were they contradictory?

Mini Glossary

Concurrent design (also known as parallel design)   Data collection for both methods is completed at the same time.

Convergence   Points of agreement.

Divergence   Points of disagreement.

Explanatory sequential   Quantitative methods are usually completed first followed by a qualitative phase.

Exploratory sequential   Qualitative methods are usually completed first followed by a quantitative phase.

Mixed-methods research   Quantitative and qualitative data collection *and* analysis methods are used in the same study to answer the research question.

Sequential design   One method is enacted before the other.

Triangulation   A concurrent mixed-methods design that combines qualitative and quantitative research methods and findings equally to answer a research question.

Mixed-Methods Shorthand

QUAL/quant   The primary or dominant study methods are qualitative.

QUANT/qual   The primary or dominant methods are quantitative.

QUAL/quant, Qual/QUANT, QUAL/QUANT   Sequential design where the qualitative methods come first.

QUANT/qual, Quant/QUAL, QUANT/QUAL   Sequential design where the quantitative methods come first.

QUANT(qual)   Qualitative methods are embedded in quantitative methodology.

QUAL(quant)   Quantitative methods are embedded in qualitative methodology.

QUANT + QUAL   or   QUAL + QUANT   Concurrent sequencing, with the qualitative and quantitative methods enacted at the same.

Key Resources

Creswell, J.W. and Plano Clark, V.L. (2017). *Designing and Conducting Mixed Methods Research*. London: Sage publications.

Heyvaert, M., Hannes, K., Maes, B., and Onghena, P. (2013). Critical appraisal of mixed methods studies. *Journal of Mixed Methods Research* 7 (4): 302–327. https://doi.org/10.1177/1558689813479449.

Moorley, C., and Cathala, X. (2019). How to appraise mixed methods research. *Evidence-Based Nursing*, 22 (2): 38–41.

Schoonenboom, J., and Johnson, R.B. (2017). How to construct a mixed methods research design. *Kölner Zeitschrift für Soziologie und Sozialpsychologie* 69 (Suppl. 2): 107–131. https://doi.org/10.1007/s11577-017-0454-1.

A.2   BLANK KEY FACTS SHEET FOR COMPLETION

KEY FACTS

Full citation: ....

Quick overview of the study: ....
....
....

Research aims or questions as stated: ....
....

Research design and why this was used:

What I think are the strengths of the research:

What I think may be its limitations:

EDECA Appraisal Considerations

Ethics

Design

Enrol

Collect

Analyse

Mini Glossary (or Terms I Don't Understand)

Resources I Need to Help Me Appraise This Paper

A.3 BLANK DJES SHEET FOR COMPLETION

Appraising (delete as appropriate) ETHICS/DESIGN/ENROL/COLLECT/ANALYSE

Study reference:

Describe ✎ What did they do?	**Justify** ⚙ Why did they do it?	**Evaluate** ⚖ Why does this matter? How does it strengthen/limit the study?	**Support** ▭ What sources have informed your points?

Now use your notes above to create an analytical appraisal point

REFERENCES

Chhabra, J., Li, W., and McDermott, B. (2022). Predictive factors for depression and anxiety in men during the perinatal period: a mixed methods study. *American Journal of Men's Health* 16 (1): 15579883221079489. https://doi.org/10.1177/15579883221079489.

Coppola, S., Miao, A.F., Allmendinger, C., and Zhang, W. (2017). Art in occupational therapy education: an exploratory mixed-methods study of an arts-based module. *Open Journal of Occupational Therapy* 5 (4): https://doi.org/10.15453/2168–6408.1320.

Creswell, J.W. and Plano Clark, V.L. (2017). *Designing and conducting mixed methods research*. London: Sage publications.

Goutaudier, N., Lopez, A., Séjourné, N. et al. (2011). Premature birth: subjective and psychological experiences in the first weeks following childbirth, a mixed-methods study. *Journal of Reproductive and Infant Psychology* 29 (4): 364–373. https://doi.org/10.1080/02646838.2011.623227.

Moorley, C. and Cathala, X. (2019). How to appraise mixed methods research. *Evidence-based Nursing* 22 (2): 38–41.

Index

Critical Appraisal Skills for Healthcare Students: A Practical Guide to Writing Evidence-based Practice Assignments, First Edition. Charlotte J. Whiffin, Donna Barnes, and Lorraine Henshaw.
© 2024 John Wiley & Sons Ltd. Published 2024 by John Wiley & Sons Ltd.